P.E.T.S.

Primary Education Thinking Skills - 1 Curriculum

Jody Nichols, Sally Thomson, Margaret Wolfe, Dodie Merritt
Illustrated by Dodie Merritt

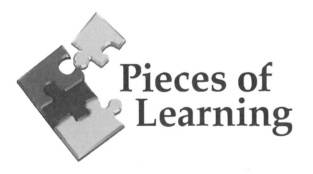
Pieces of Learning

CLC0199
ISBN 978-1-880505-24-3
Cover Design by John Steele
© Illustrations by Dodie Merritt
Graphic Production by Pamela Pirk
© 1997 Pieces of Learning
www.piecesoflearning.com
Marion IL 62959

Printed by McNaughton & Gunn, Inc.
Saline MI U.S.A.
05/2010

Table of Contents

Acknowledgments

The authors of this book would like to thank the administration of Illinois School Districts #47 and #424 for their support of the P.E.T.S. program as well as the many primary teachers in whose classes these materials were field-tested. Also many thanks to our families for their support.

A special thanks to Ryan Arens, Devin Beggs, Jami Biedermann, Travis Brown, Kelly Chrystal, Jessica Doerrfeld, Grainger Greene, Lindsey Hines, Alaine Lecuyer, Felicia Lee, Keith McKenna, Adam McNerney, Mark Meador, Morgan Meredith, Drew Nystrom, Jessica Ocheskey, Josh Osborn, Sarah Pierce, Heidi Quinn, Kierstyn Rauch, Evan Schano, Chris Schroeder, Becca Terdich, Christina Werderitch, Brynn Wolford and Tim Yaguchi for the contribution of their artwork to "Laboratory Limpets" and "Sybil's Creatures."

PETS™ (Primary Education Thinking Skills)

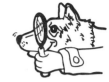

Dudley the Detective

DEFINITION

. . . is a systematized enrichment and diagnostic thinking skills program that can be easily integrated into an existing primary curriculum. P.E.T.S.™ serves the dual purpose of helping in the identification of academically talented students and teaching students higher level thinking skills.

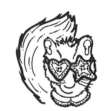

Isabel the Inventor

PROGRAM RATIONALE

P.E.T.S.™ follows the taxonomy outlined by Benjamin Bloom, presenting lessons in analysis, synthesis, and evaluation. These higher order skills are less emphasized in most primary curricula, yet students of all ability levels have shown interest in and understanding of these different types of thinking.

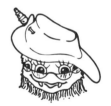

Sybil the Scientist

P.E.T.S.™ also provides teachers with the opportunity to identify talented students early in their school careers and to implement a curriculum which will best suit their special needs. This identification occurs in the classroom setting.

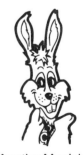

Yolanda the Yarnspinner

The format of the P.E.T.S.™ delivery system follows a modification of the Triad Model posed by Dr. Joseph Renzulli. The entire class is given the opportunity to experience the challenge of the new thinking skill. Based on teacher observation and student interest, a small group of students is then given further opportunity to explore the thinking skill in a variety of in-depth activities. During the small group activities, the teacher is able to evaluate student potential further and to plan student programming accordingly.

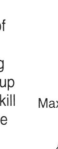

Max the Magician

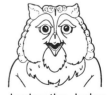

Jordan the Judge

PROGRAM OVERVIEW

P.E.T.S.™ has a two-tier delivery system which is easily facilitated by the classroom teacher or a visiting specialist. The first tier focuses on whole class enrichment activities for the entire grade level population. The second tier activities are used in small group settings to challenge the more capable students.

At the beginning of each of the six units, a character from P.E.T.S.™ introduces a high level thinking skill used in his or her job.

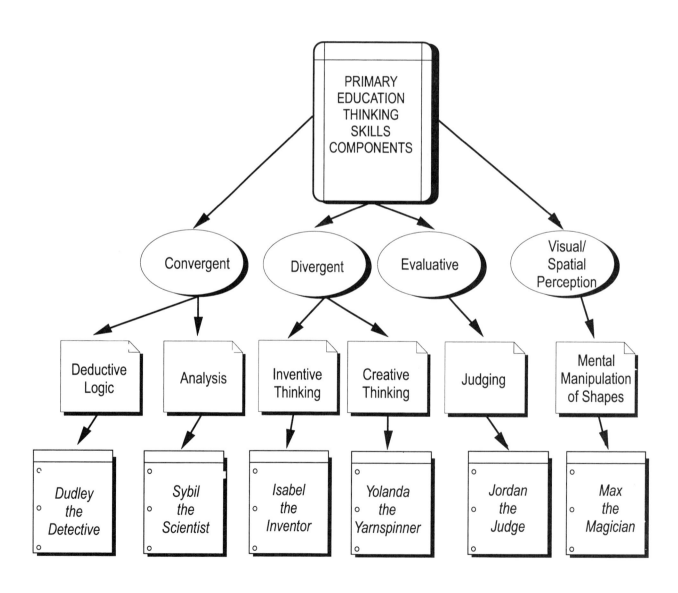

Each character serves as a guide through a story to introduce the type of thinking and a series of whole class activities to reinforce the type of thinking. Imaginative memory triggers are included with each introductory lesson.

Dudley the Dectective - a detective badge
Isabel the Inventor - Brainfocals™
Sybil the Scientist - magnifying glass

Yolanda the Yarnspinner - bookmark
Max the Magician - pencil holder
Jordan the Judge - gavel

Additional activities are provided for small group sessions. These activities stimulate students with high interest, challenging exercises, many of which are hands-on. Detailed lesson plans are provided for all whole class and small group lessons. An *Ask Me What I Did Today* prompt is included with each unit to be sent home with students who participated in the small group.

Parallel to the instructional element of P.E.T.S.™ is a two-tier diagnostic tool for identifying talented students. A behavioral checklist that is used by the classroom teacher during the whole group activities provides information about students who show potential. Students who show outstanding aptitude during the whole class lessons, as recorded on the checklist, are invited to participate in the small group sessions. A more detailed checklist is used during the small group sessions to better identify student levels of talent and abilities.

The P.E.T.S .™ program is comprised of:

— twelve lessons for the whole class

— twelve activities for the small groups

— detailed lesson plans

— diagnostic checklists

— six *Ask Me What I Did Today* prompts

IDENTIFYING TALENTED LEARNERS

The primary classroom teacher has a very diverse population in both maturity and intellect. Some students will immediately appear talented in certain areas and other students need to be given opportunities to show their abilities. Before attempting to use the checklists, teachers need to understand the different characteristics and behaviors which indicate that a student might be talented in a particular area.

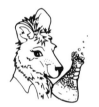

DIVERGENT THINKING

Those students who excel at divergent thinking are able to list many responses to questions or brainstorm many ideas. Not only are they fluent in their thinking but are also very flexible. They tend to be original, giving off-beat and sometimes very humorous responses. These students can elaborate or expand upon an idea and because of this the flow of ideas may be interrupted. An advanced vocabulary is sometimes displayed during the divergent thinking activities.

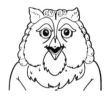

CONVERGENT THINKING

The ability to intuitively see the correct answer is one characteristic of students who excel at deductive/ convergent thinking. They tend to see the interrelationships between clues and defer judgment until all clues have been collected. Many times they will display outside knowledge about a topic that will help them discover the correct solution.

EVALUATIVE THINKING

The students who are able to evaluate and offer a solution that is based on valid considerations have an opportunity to shine during these specially designed lessons. The checklists support behaviors such as seeing more than one viewpoint, understanding considerations, and supporting decisions and opinions.

VISUAL/SPATIAL PERCEPTION

These students demonstrate a good memory for detail. They may not be as verbal as their classmates and therefore may not have as much opportunity to demonstrate their talents during traditional classroom activities. These students often enjoy activities involving hands-on building of three-dimensional objects from two-dimensional drawings. During class work, these students often respond best to visual images such as graphic organizers and instructional computer programs.

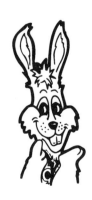

IDENTIFYING TALENTED LEARNERS
DURING WHOLE CLASS LESSONS

The P.E.T.S.™ program can help both classroom and specialty teachers identify talented students in whole class situations and small group situations. The whole class lessons are the first tier in identifying students. The ideal situation is to have two teachers in the classroom, one teacher presenting the thinking skill lesson and one teacher observing students' behaviors. If two teachers are not available, the program will work with a parent volunteer or a teacher's aide. If this is the case, the teacher can help the aide by using key phrases to indicate that a student's name should be added to the checklist. For example a teacher may say, *"Wow, Julie, that's a great way to use an earlier clue to see the new clue."*

Six behavior characteristics have been included for each thinking skill. These behaviors vary from thinking skill to thinking skill. Checklists are provided in each unit as an easy reference for teachers. As a student is observed showing one of the behaviors the teacher records the student's name in the appropriate box. If the student shows additional behaviors in that category, the teacher can add check marks after the name. To differentiate between sessions, record each lesson's responses in a different color.

It is important for the teacher observing students to look beyond just the most vocal students who are the first to answer. All students need to be observed and questioned to give all students an opportunity to show their potential. There is a category on the Behavioral Checklist to indicate students who show outstanding performance on seat work or class work. The Behavioral Checklists include an opportunity to list students who were not present during the thinking skill lesson or have shown the characteristics in other classroom situations.

It is essential for the teacher to remember that the number of talented learners in any one classroom may be quite small. The P.E.T.S.™ program has been designed to identify this small population; do not expect the entire class to achieve mastery of the lessons. All students will benefit from exposure to these higher-level thinking skills, but the actual number of students demonstrating mastery level may be quite small. That's OK.

At the end of one or two whole class thinking skill lessons, the students who are talented in that type of thinking will stand out as the teacher examines the Behavioral Checklist. The students frequently listed on the Behavioral Checklist and listed in a variety of areas are the students who are invited to the small group lessons. The small group may vary from thinking skill to thinking skill.

IDENTIFYING TALENTED LEARNERS
DURING SMALL GROUP LESSONS

The second tier of the identification process is the small group lessons. The small group may consist of students from a variety of classrooms or a group from the same classroom.

The small group lessons are designed to provide further enrichment and opportunities for teachers to observe additional behaviors that identify talented students. Lesson plans are provided for the small group lessons. The lesson plans reflect the faster pace delivery and in depth content appropriate for gifted students. The small group lessons are not as structured as the whole class lessons and provide students with more opportunities for interaction and cooperative problem solving. These lessons are intended to be diagnostic as opposed to instructional.

Use the form on the following page during the small group lessons for record keeping and note taking about students.

NOTES

PETS™ Small Group Checklist
A Cumulative Student Record

STUDENT:　　　　　　　　　　　　　　**SCHOOL:**　　　　　　　**TEACHER:**

GRADE LEVEL:

		CONVERGENT				DIVERGENT				VISUAL/ SPATIAL		EVALUA- TIVE	
		Deductive		Analytical		Inventive		Creative					

YEAR:　　　　　　**DATE**

ACTIVITY

+　　　**✓**　　　**–**

CHARACTERISTICS													
Does difficult mental tasks													
Retains information													
Comprehends concepts													
Sees inter-relationships													
Reasons independently													
Makes evaluations													
Reads above grade level													
Uses an extensive vocabulary													
Enjoys puzzles/problems with a twist													
Uses alternative methods to solve problems													
Displays an advanced sense of humor													
Exhibits curiosity													
Demonstrates leadership													
Is fluent with ideas													
Shows flexibility													
Exhibits originality													
Elaborates with many details													
Demonstrates task commitment													

COMMENTS:

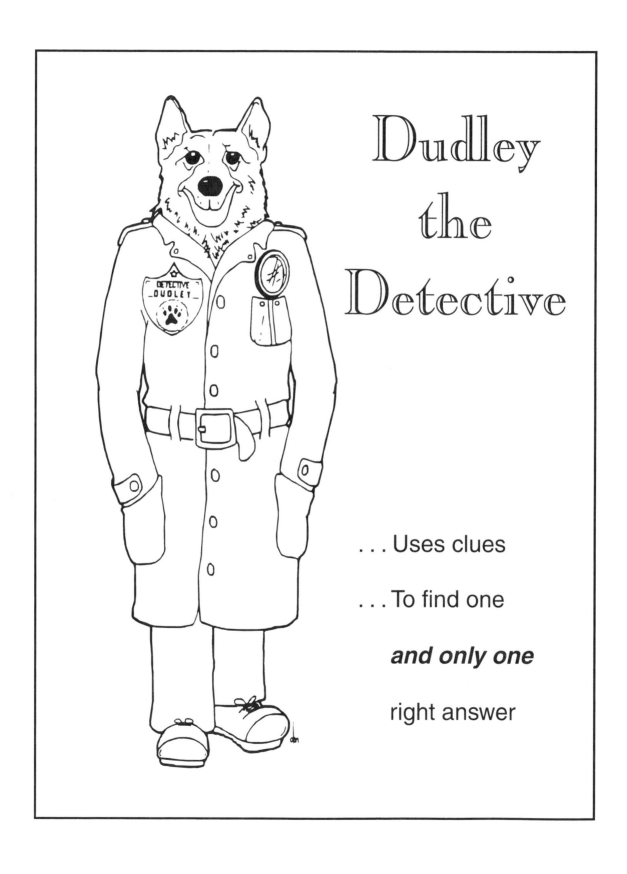

Dudley the Detective

. . . Uses clues

. . . To find one

and only one

right answer

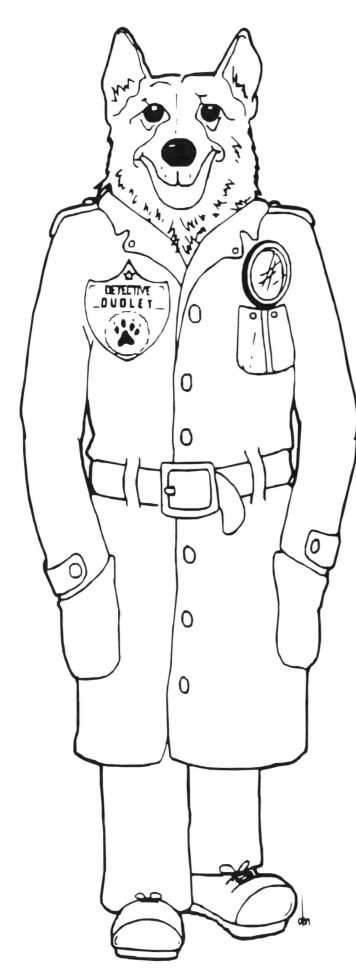

Dudley the Detective

. . . Uses clues

. . . To find one

and only one

right answer

Convergent / Deductive Thinking

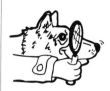

DETECTIVE THINKING
WHOLE CLASS
LESSON 1

PURPOSE

The purpose of this lesson is to introduce the students to **deductive/convergent thinking**. The students will be introduced to *Dudley the Detective* who puts his clues together to arrive at the one correct answer to the problem. The students should be made to understand that in deductive/convergent thinking:

— There is one and only one right answer.
— They may need to put together many pieces of information in order to find the one right answer.
— They may feel like saying *"I have it!"* when they find the answer.
— They may not see the answer right away and need to reflect on some of the clues.
— Patience is important in not jumping to conclusions and in reflecting on clues.

TEACHER MATERIALS

— one copy of the *Dudley the Detective* story to read aloud to the students
— an overhead transparency of the picture of *Dudley the Detective* and /or a class set of duplicated pictures for the students to color
— a duplicated class set of detective badges, perhaps run on yellow or goldenrod paper
— pins or masking tape for the badges
— a *Mystery Creatures* story to read to the students
— an overhead and duplicated class set of *Mystery Creatures* worksheets
— a duplicated class set of the Challenge pages *Who is Mary?* and *Which Dog Belongs to Mary?*
— Behavioral Checklist - *Detective Thinking*

STUDENT MATERIALS

— crayons or markers
— pencils
— scissors

LESSON PLAN

1. Introduce the lesson by asking students if they know what a *detective* is. Brainstorm with students some detectives they know and what those detectives do.

2. Tell the students that today they are going to meet *Dudley the Detective* who thinks in a very special way. Using the overhead projector, show them the picture (page 12) of Dudley. You may wish to have them color the picture of Dudley (page 13) at this time or following the reading of the story.

3. Read the *Dudley the Detective* story.

4. Review with the students these points from the story:

  — In deductive thinking, there is only one right answer. All the students should arrive at the same answer to be considered correct.
  — The students may feel like saying *"Aha!"* or *"I have it!"* when they find the right answer.
  — Reflecting or delaying judgment of certain information is necessary.
  — It is often necessary to put more than one clue together in order to find the needed information to solve the problem.
  — Patience is important. Avoid jumping to conclusions or relying on pre-conceived notions.

5. Help the students cut out and make detective badges, the memory trigger for this unit. Have them wear them while doing the deductive activities. They should label the badges with their names or choose a creative *detective name* if you prefer.

6. Distribute *Mystery Creatures* worksheets. While wearing their badges, have the students listen to the *Mystery Creatures* story. Following the clues outlined in the story, students should draw in the boxes on their worksheets the creatures they think are being described. Remind them that these are REAL creatures, and fantasy drawings should be avoided.

ANSWER KEY   to *Mystery Creatures*   1. turtle   2. owl   3. bear   4. fox

CHALLENGE PAGES

Who is Mary?
Which Dog Belongs to Mary?

7. Distribute the Challenge Pages to students. You may need to read the clues aloud to non-reading students. If students have the reading ability, the Challenge Pages can be assigned as independent work. If the Challenge pages are going to be used for assessing student potential, it is important that students work individually.

DIAGNOSTIC NOTES

During this lesson, the teacher and observer will be looking for students who display specific characteristics. Those students will then be invited to the small group sessions for additional activities. Some teachers explain the structure of the **Primary Education Thinking Skills** curriculum to the students before actually starting the lessons. During the explanation, the teacher might point out to students the importance of volunteering during the lessons. This is the main opportunity for the teachers to know what students are thinking and students need to share their thoughts.

Characteristic behaviors and responses are listed on a checklist, one checklist for each of the six units. There is an overlap of characteristics among the units. The following is a short summary of what to look for in student behaviors and responses for the Detective Thinking Unit.

GRASPS CONCEPTS QUICKLY - Look for students who are able to quickly understand and use the process of elimination. List the students who are the first to figure out the correct answers.

DRAWS RELATIONSHIPS BETWEEN THE LESSON AND OUTSIDE INFORMATION Look for students who exhibit knowledge from outside the classroom and use it as an additional clue in solving the puzzle. After the lesson is over, students should be noted who see the relationship between convergent thinking and other classroom activities.

INTUITIVELY SEES ANSWERS - Some students who are excellent convergent thinkers are unable to verbalize how they figured out the answer. Note students when this occurs.

SEES AN INTERRELATIONSHIP OF CLUES - Look for students who see how to build one clue's information on a previous clue to deduce the answer.

ABLE TO DEFER JUDGMENT - Look for students who are willing to wait until they have figured out the correct answer. These students avoid guessing until they determine the correct answer.

DISPLAYS A LONG ATTENTION SPAN - In addition to a long attention span, look for students who want to work on convergent type activities. An enthusiasm towards this type of problem usually indicates an ability to solve the problems.

Who is Mary? and ***Which Dog Belongs to Mary?***
Look for students who are able to solve the puzzles correctly.

PETS

List names of students as each behavior appears.
 	
   Add checkmarks after name if behavior is repeated.
 	
   Use a different color of ink or pencil for each whole group lesson.
	Behavioral Checklist
	----------- 	
	Detective Thinking
	(Deductive Logic/Convergent)
		Teacher _____
		Grade: 1 ___ 2 ___ 3 ___
		
		Dates of whole 1. _____
		group instruction: 2. _____

GRASPS CONCEPTS VERY QUICKLY	USES ONE CLUE TO DETERMINE ANOTHER OR PUTS CLUES TOGETHER -- *SEES INTERRELATIONSHIP OF CLUES*
DRAWS RELATIONSHIPS BETWEEN LESSON AND OUTSIDE INFORMATION TO HELP DETERMINE CONCLUSIONS	GATHERS AND WEIGHS ALL INFORMATION BEFORE DECIDING ON AN ANSWER -- *DEFERS JUDGMENT*
INTUITIVELY SEES ANSWERS WITHOUT INTERMEDIATE STEPS	*DISPLAYS LONG ATTENTION SPAN* -- WORKS EXERCISE DILIGENTLY TO THE END
PETS classwork indicates an outstanding ability to use this thinking skill.	The following student/s did not participate during the thinking skills lessons, but I see these behaviors during **regular class time.**

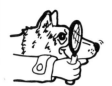

Dudley The Detective

One bright sunny morning, Dudley the Detective woke up, stretched, and yawned.

"What a *great* morning," he said. "This will be a fine day for solving a mystery."

Dudley was a detective. He *loved* to solve mysteries. Dudley thought the best way to spend a morning was to **look for clues** and **gather information** about the latest mystery.

Dudley's favorite afternoon was spent **thinking** about all the information he had gathered. He was always careful **not to jump to conclusions** quickly. He preferred to ponder the mystery until after dinner.

Once Dudley had eaten dinner, the phone would begin to ring, for all the people in town knew that Dudley would have figured out the *one* correct answer to the mystery. Dudley usually figured out the correct answer while washing dishes. He would exclaim loudly, *"I've got it!"*

This particular morning, as Dudley stretched and yawned, he remembered, with some disappointment, that he did not have a mystery to solve today. Although disappointed, he put on his detective uniform anyway.

He put on his trench coat, since many detectives wear trench coats. Dudley also put his magnifying glass in his coat pocket. Detectives need magnifying glasses to search carefully for clues.

The only thing Dudley needed now to be ready for a mystery was his detective badge. Dudley had received this very special badge at detective school because he had shown what great detective thinking he used.

As Dudley looked around the room, he could not find his detective badge. He looked high. He looked low. He looked left. He looked right. He looked *everywhere* but he could not find his detective badge.

This distressed Dudley the Detective, but then he remembered he was the *best* detective in town, and if anyone could find his detective badge, *he* could.

The first thing he needed to do was to **look for clues**. Dudley noticed that the window was open. He also saw muddy paw prints that appeared to be those of a raccoon. Dudley knew that Rascal Raccoon often got into trouble, but Dudley did not want to jump to the wrong conclusion, so he continued looking for clues.

Outside, Dudley noticed more paw prints going up and over the fence toward Rascal Raccoon's house. As Dudley was standing outside looking for clues with his magnifying glass, he had to shade his eyes from the bright sun reflecting off the apple tree in his backyard. After looking all over the yard and back inside the house, Dudley had not found any more clues.

After lunch, Dudley sat down to think about the case.

He thought it seemed like Rascal Raccoon was the culprit, but Dudley knew he **should not jump to a quick conclusion.**

Dudley continued to ponder the mystery during dinner, and as he was washing the dishes, he shouted, *"I've got it!"*

(At this time you may choose to ask for student responses.)

Do you think you've got it?

Dudley got a ladder and went out to the apple tree. He climbed up to the spot from which the sunlight had been reflecting so brightly into his eyes earlier that day.

Sure enough, there in Rosalyn Robin's nest was Dudley's detective badge. Rosalyn Robin admitted to seeing the beautiful shiny object in Dudley's house and to flying in that open window to take the detective badge.

Rascal Raccoon had been in Dudley's house, too, but not to take the detective badge. That was a mystery that Dudley would save until tomorrow.

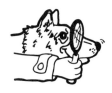

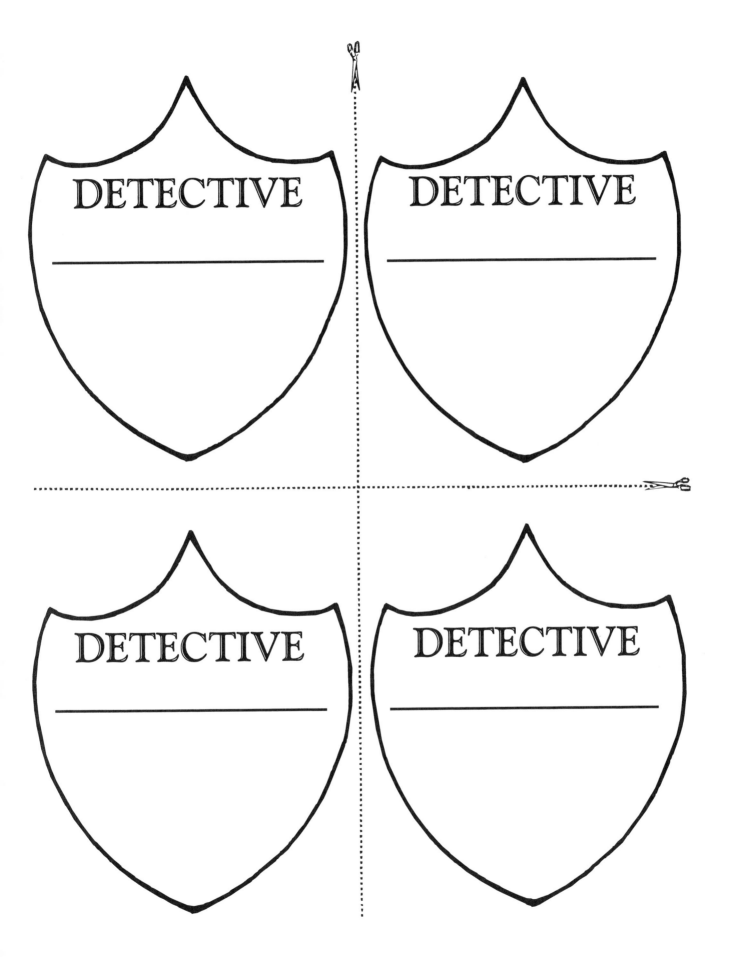

MYSTERY CREATURES

Dudley, Rosalyn Robin, and their friends in Crystal Pond Woods have another mystery for you to solve. Here are descriptions of four real animals. Three are friends and live in the woods. The fourth one is a mysterious stranger. Listen to the clues and help Dudley figure out who is who by drawing what you think these creatures look like.

1. My favorite afternoons are spent sunning on a log by the pond. When Rascal Raccoon comes by, I ignore him by pulling my head, tail, and four feet into "my house."

2. Some say I am very wise. Maybe that's because when I'm not flying I can turn my head almost all the way around. I don't miss much. I'm also forever asking one question.

3. My love for honey sometimes gets me into a whole lot of trouble. When I stick my paw into the beehive, I usually get stung on my black nose. My brown fur helps to protect me everywhere else.

4. I'm afraid Rosalyn Robin spotted me last night sneaking through the woods. I'm sure she noticed my pointy ears and long red bushy tail. I know she does not feel safe while I'm around. She needn't worry — even though my legs are short, I can travel very quickly, and I'll be gone by dawn.

Name _____

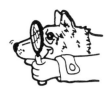

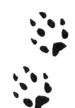

Mystery Creatures

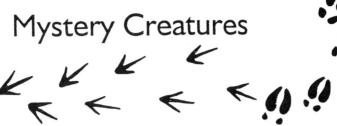

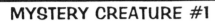

MYSTERY CREATURE #1	MYSTERY CREATURE #2
NAME _____	NAME _____

MYSTERY CREATURE #3	MYSTERY CREATURE #4
NAME _____	NAME _____

Name _____

Who Is Mary?

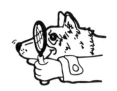

Dudley is looking for Mary. Use these clues to help you find Mary. Color her.

1. Mary has long hair.

2. Mary does **not** play with dolls.

3. Mary is happy.

4. Mary likes to skate.

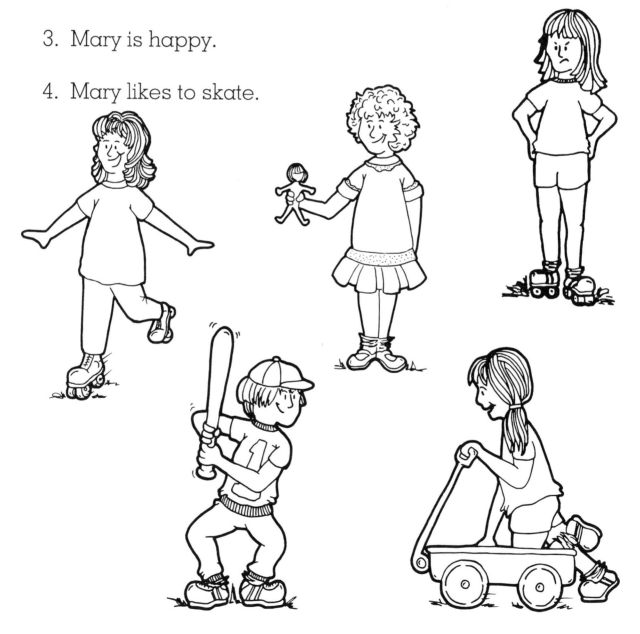

Name _____

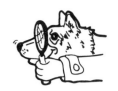

Which Dog Belongs To Mary?

Use these clues to help you find Mary's dog. Color it.

1. Its tail is long.

2. It is **not** a big dog.

3. It does **not** have spots.

4. Its ears are like its tail.

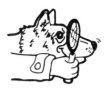

DETECTIVE THINKING
WHOLE CLASS
LESSON 2

PURPOSE

The purpose of this lesson is for students to review and reinforce the concepts of **deductive thinking.** Students will look for clues in a picture and deduce correct answers to a series of questions. Students should be reminded that:

— There is one and only one right answer.
— They may need to put together many pieces of information in order to find the one right answer.
— They may feel like saying *"I have it!"* when they find the answer.
— They may need to reflect on some of the clues since they may not see the answer right away.
— They need to refrain from jumping to conclusions.

TEACHER MATERIALS

— an overhead transparency of *A Party in the Woods*
— an overhead transparency of *Lost Toys*
— an overhead transparency of *Who Gets Which Gift?*
— one duplicated class set of *Ladybug Leap*
— one duplicated class set of *Color the Flowers*
— Behavioral Checklist - *Detective Thinking*

STUDENT MATERIALS

— crayons
— pencils

LESSON PLAN

1. Review with students the concepts introduced with Dudley the Detective in Lesson 1. Discuss with students the characteristics of a *detective.*

2. Tell students that they are going to be detectives today. Put a copy of *A Party in the Woods* on the overhead projector. Give students an opportunity to study the scene before discussing the picture. This scene has pictures of most of the main characters in the P.E.T.S.™ program. During this lesson, it might be helpful to use the name of each

character. The owl is *Jordan the Judge*, the kangaroo is *Sybil the Scientist*, the squirrel is *Isabel the Inventor*, and the rabbit is *Max the Magician.*

3. The following are questions the teacher should ask students as they study *A Party in the Woods.* The questions do not have to be asked in order. The discussion can evolve as students make observations and inferences based on the clues. The answers are provided in italics. As students give you answers, ask them what they see to support their conclusions.

DISCUSSION QUESTIONS

— What celebration is going on here? *(A birthday party.)*
— How can you tell? *(There is a cake with candles and a pile of presents. The candles on the cake is the key clue since it is the only celebration that has candles on a cake.)*
— Whose birthday is it? How can you tell? *(The owl's, Jordan the Judge, because he is by the cake, the cake has many candles, and one of the presents has "owl" attached. Students may say it is the bear's birthday since the bear is next to the cake, but that is the only evidence that supports the bear.)*
— What season is it? *(It is autumn because there are only a few leaves left on the trees, there are leaves on the ground, and it is warm enough to not need a coat.)*
— Someone at the party is named Bill. Who do you think it is? Why? *(He is the boy with the fishing pole. His name is on his shirt but only "LL" is visible.)*
— What do you think Bill is going to do at the party? Why? *(He has a fishing pole, and there is a pond with a fish in it so he is probably going fishing.)*
— Sybil the Scientist has just arrived at the party. What do you think her present might be? Why? *(The present might be soft or something curved. It is also light enough to carry. Accept any reasonable answers which fit.)*
— What other things are going on at the party? *(It appears that Max the Magician is putting on a magic show. Some of the other things brought up by students can be accepted if they are supported by clues or evidence in the picture.)*

4. After completing the discussion, put the overhead transparencies of *Lost Toys* and *Who Gets Which Gift?* on the overhead projector. Work through the activities as a class.

ANSWERS

Lost Toys -   1. Brad 2. Bill 3. Betty 4. Brenda 5. Beth
Who Gets Which Gift? -   Isabel, Max, Yolanda, Dudley, Jordan
                            Jordan gets the biggest gift.

Ladybug Leap
Color the Flowers

5. Distribute the Challenge Pages to students. Teachers may need to read the clues aloud to non-reading students. If students have the reading ability, the Challenge Pages can be assigned as independent work. If the Challenge Pages are going to be used for assessing student potential, it is important that students work individually.

DIAGNOSTIC NOTES

Characteristic behaviors and responses are listed on a checklist, one checklist for each of the six units. There is an overlap of characteristics among the units. The following is a short summary of what to look for in student behaviors and responses for the Detective Thinking Unit.

GRASPS CONCEPTS QUICKLY - Look for students who are able to quickly understand and use the process of elimination. List the students who are the first to figure out the correct answers.

DRAWS RELATIONSHIPS BETWEEN THE LESSON AND OUTSIDE INFORMATION
Look for students who exhibit knowledge from outside the classroom and use it as an additional clue in solving the puzzle. After the lesson is over, students should be noted who see the relationship between convergent thinking and other classroom activities.

INTUITIVELY SEES ANSWERS - Some students who are excellent convergent thinkers are unable to verbalize how they figured out the answer. Note students when this occurs.

SEES AN INTERRELATIONSHIP OF CLUES - Look for students who see how to build one clue's information on a previous clue to deduce the answer.

ABLE TO DEFER JUDGMENT - Look for students who are willing to wait until they have figured out the correct answer. These students avoid guessing until they determine the correct answer.

DISPLAYS A LONG ATTENTION SPAN - In addition to a long attention span, look for students who want to work on convergent type activities. An enthusiasm towards this type of problem usually indicates an ability to solve the problems.

Ladybug Leap and ***Color the Flowers***
Look for students who are able to correctly solve the puzzles.
Ladybug Leap: (1) 9   (2) 15   (3) 6   (4) 2   (5) 12
Color the Flowers: (l-r) purple, yellow, orange, blue, red

A Party In The Woods

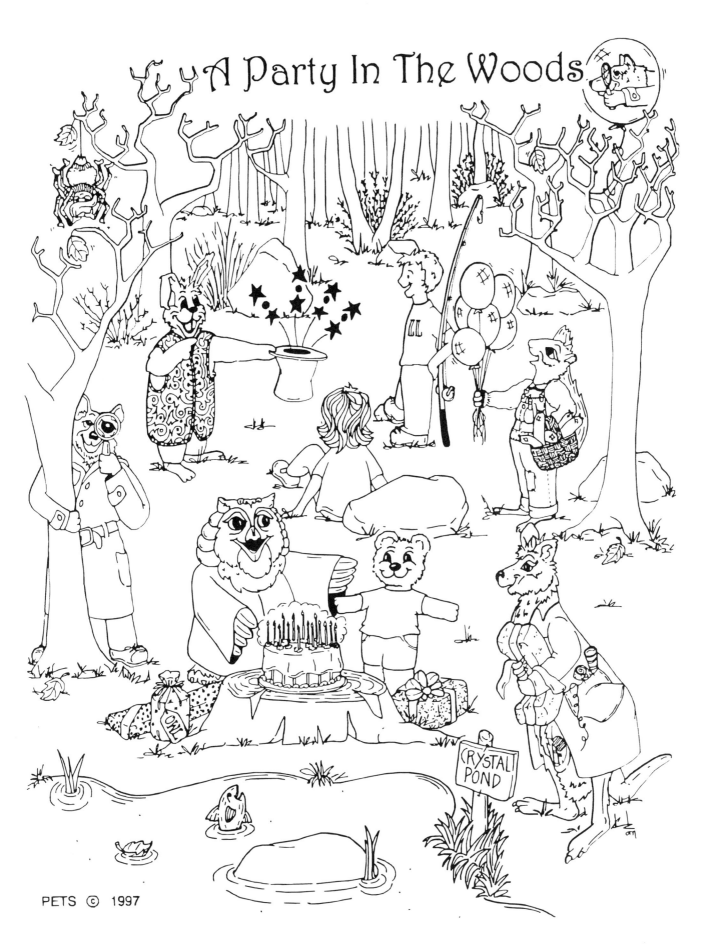

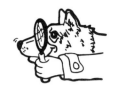

Lost Toys

Dudley found some lost toys in Crystal Pond Woods. He wants to return them to the rightful owners. Read all the clues and write the owner's name by each toy.

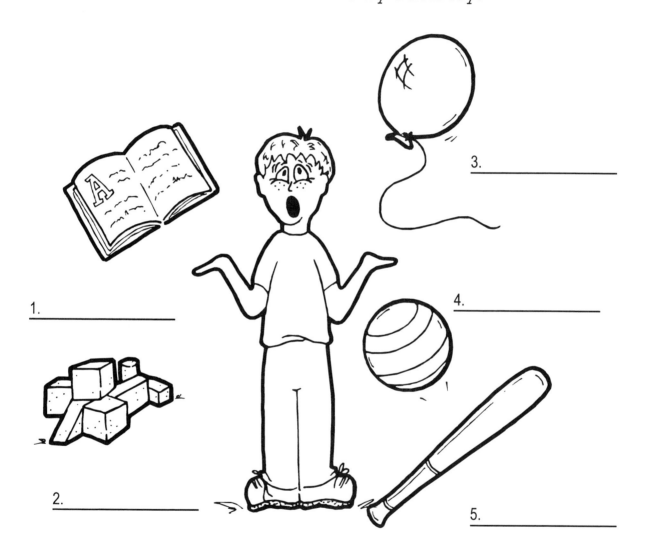

3. _____

1. _____

4. _____

2. _____

5. _____

1. Betty does not play with balls.

2. Bill likes to build with blocks.

3. Beth's toy is **not** round.

4. Brenda has a toy.

5. Brad loves to read.

Name _____

Who Gets Which Gift?

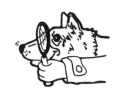

Write the proper names on the gift tags.

1. Max's gift is

   not on top.

2. Yolanda gets the gift

   right below Max's.

3. Dudley's gift is

   long and thin.

4. Jordan gets a gift.

5. Isabel's gift has

   two bows.

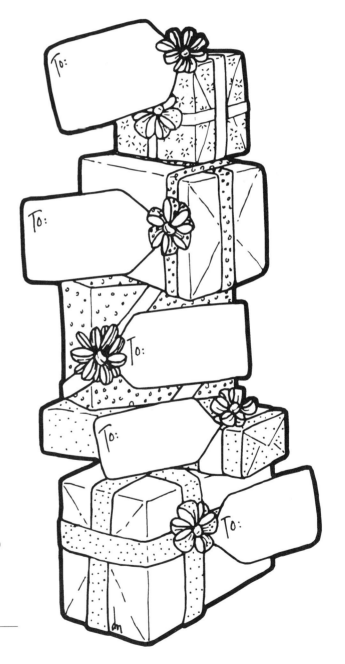

Who gets the biggest gift?

_____

Ladybug Leap

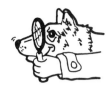

Five ladybugs are racing to the tip of the leaf. Put the correct number of spots on the back of each ladybug. Write the number of spots on the line by each ladybug.

1. The 15-spotted ladybug came in second.

2. The 6-spotted ladybug did not finish last.

3. The 12-spotted one finished right behind the one with 2 spots.

4. The 9-spotted ladybug is the fastest.

5. The last 3 ladybugs have even numbers of spots.

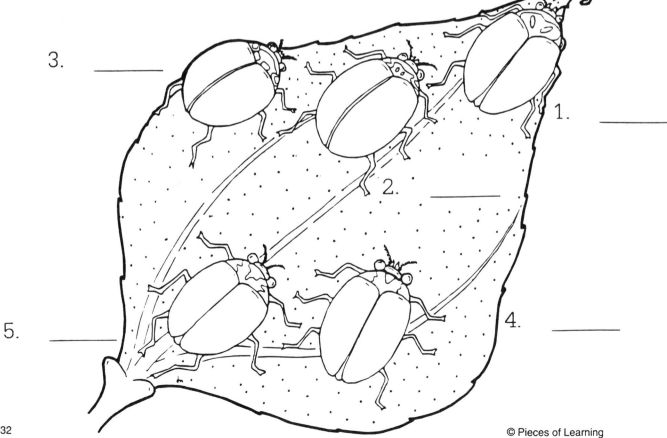

Name _____

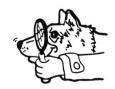

Color The Flowers

Use these clues to help color the flowers in Crystal Pond Woods.

1. The biggest flower is yellow.

2. The blue flower is not on the end.

3. The orange flower is between the yellow one and the blue one.

4. One flower is purple.

5. The smallest flower is red.

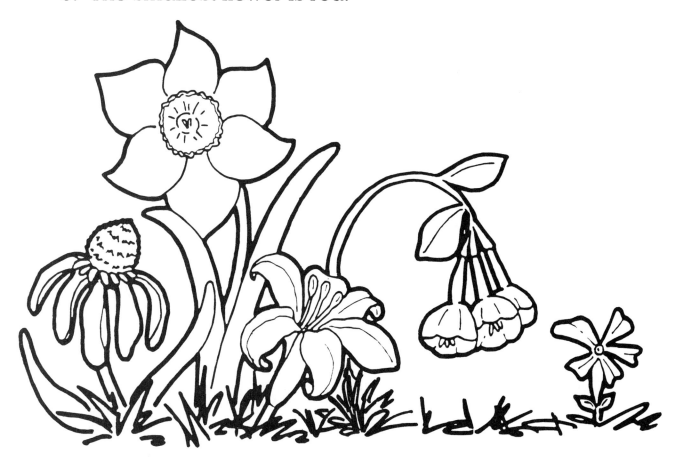

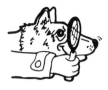

DETECTIVE THINKING
SMALL GROUP
LESSON 1

PURPOSE

The purpose of this lesson is to give students an opportunity to practice **deductive thinking.** Students will be using the attribute blocks. During the lesson, the teacher will be observing and assessing students as one means of identifying potentially talented learners.

TEACHER MATERIALS

— a group set of *Can you find your way through Crystal Pond Woods?*

STUDENT MATERIALS

— a set of attribute blocks – commercial sets are available. Directions are provided for making sets. A master copy of the shapes is also provided.

LESSON PLAN

1. Spread sets of attribute blocks on a table, one set in front of each student. The teacher needs to secretly take one block and hide it. Take a different block from each student's set so they each have to figure out the solution.

2. Introduce the word *ATTRIBUTE*. Discuss that attributes are characteristics of something. Ask students what are some characteristics or attributes about themselves. Students' characteristics may include hair color, eye color, height, gender, etc., but should not include what they are wearing. Discuss why not. Then ask students to determine the characteristics of the attribute blocks.

Attributes of the blocks, which should be suggested by the students are:

    size -   big and little
    thickness-thin and thick
    color -   blue, red, or yellow
    shape -   triangle, square, hexagon, circle, rectangle

Have students hold up each shape, compare thin with thick, and compare large with small blocks of the same shape.

3. Tell students that each block has a special name of its own, which comes from naming each of its four attributes. Have students hold up their BIG, THICK, BLUE, HEXAGON. (Make sure you ask for examples which are not in the student set.)

4. Next, tell students that they are going to practice their detective thinking by solving a mystery. Tell them that you secretly took one block from each set and that you have hidden the block. Tell them that you will return the block to them if they can name it for you. They must name each of the four attributes in order to correctly name the block and get it back.

Note the processes students use in order to solve this problem. Some students may be able to visualize and determine in their heads the missing block. Other students may group the blocks to determine the missing one.

If students name an incorrect block, one which is still in their sets, simply point to the incorrect choice on the table and say, *"There is your (choice of block). If you have it on the table, I cannot have it. Try to gather more clues."*

Students may at first try to guess randomly, but they will see in time that they need to group their blocks in order to determine the missing one. Do not encourage this. Allow them to arrive at this conclusion on their own.

5. As students correctly name and receive their blocks, set each student to the next task: to build one-difference trains.

Select one block from the student's set and set it on the table in front of him/her. Name that block with the student. (This is your BIG, THIN, RED SQUARE.) Tell the student that you want them to create a train of seven more blocks behind this block for a total of eight blocks in the train. At each step the student should change only one attribute. For example, if you began the student's train with the BIG, THIN, RED SQUARE they could next place the LITTLE, THIN, RED SQUARE or the BIG, THICK, RED SQUARE or any BIG, THICK, RED SHAPE.

The third step of the train should be one attribute different from the second, and so on. When the student thinks he/she has completed the train correctly, you will check the train by asking:
    "What did you change from here to here?" (Pointing to the first and second blocks)
"And from here to here?" (Pointing to the second and third blocks) and so on down the train to the end.

If the student has placed an incorrect block, the teacher should help him/her see that they have changed too many attributes and the train should be corrected from that point. Don't have the student start over. Simply change the blocks as necessary.

6. When the student successfully completes a one-difference train, ask him/her to try a two-difference train, which is the same as a one-difference train except there are two new attributes at each step.

7. When a two-difference train has been successfully accomplished, have the students try circular trains of one-difference. At each step one attribute is changed, but the train makes a circle instead of a straight line so that the last block must also be one attribute different from the original block in the train. Two-difference circular trains may also be attempted.

8. Should anyone finish all the trains described above, have the student attempt to make a figure-eight train of one or two attribute differences. Place a block on the table, and tell the student that this is the center of a figure eight. The student should add four blocks above this one and four blocks below this one, so that when the "eight" shape is drawn, the center block is crossed going from the top of the eight to the bottom and again going back up from the bottom to the top. Each time the center block is crossed, it must have the correct number of attribute differences. This is a challenging activity for primary students.

9. Give students the worksheet *Can you find your way through Crystal Pond Woods?* Explain to students that an attribute block goes in each circle. The number of lines between the circles indicates the number of attribute changes between the circles.

DIAGNOSTIC NOTES

Some students may not be able to complete all of the activities. Students who grasp the concepts quickly and are able to move through all the activities show strong indication of being very talented in the area of deductive/convergent thinking. Students who create their own trains or designs with the attribute blocks are also indicating high potential.

NOTES

Attribute Blocks

Student sets of attribute blocks can be made by cutting out the shapes found on the next page. These sets will have three (3) attributes: shape, size, and color.

To add the color attribute, color one of each different shape red, one blue, and one yellow. These sets will each contain thirty (30) blocks, one each of the following:

large blue rectangle	large yellow rectangle	small red rectangle
large blue square	large yellow square	small red square
large blue circle	large yellow circle	small red circle
large blue triangle	large yellow triangle	small red triangle
large blue hexagon	large yellow hexagon	small red hexagon
large red rectangle	small blue rectangle	small yellow rectangle
large red square	small blue square	small yellow square
large red circle	small blue circle	small yellow circle
large red triangle	small blue triangle	small yellow triangle
large red hexagon	small blue hexagon	small yellow hexagon

For greater durability: Laminate pages after the shapes have been colored before they are cut out; and/or glue pages onto poster board before the shapes are cut out.

Commercial sets of attribute blocks have four (4) attributes: shape, size, color, and thickness. These sets contain sixty (60) blocks.

To add the thickness attribute to the above student sets, glue two sheets of poster board together plus the page of shapes for the thick blocks, and use one thickness of poster board and the shapes page for the thin blocks.

It is recommended that poster board block pieces be laminated to help thick pieces stay together and to keep pieces clean and in good shape.

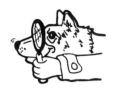

An Attribute Blocks Set To Make

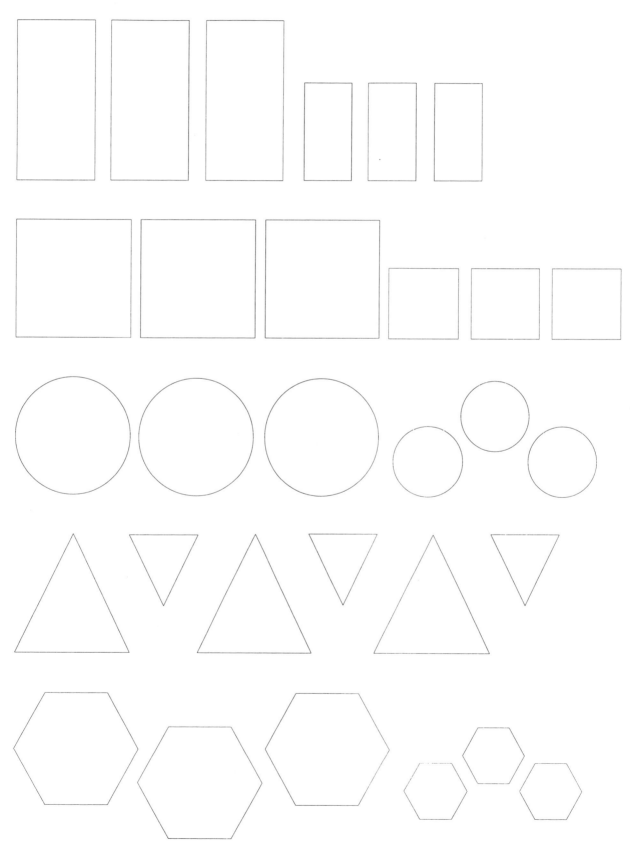

Can you find your way through Crystal Pond Woods?

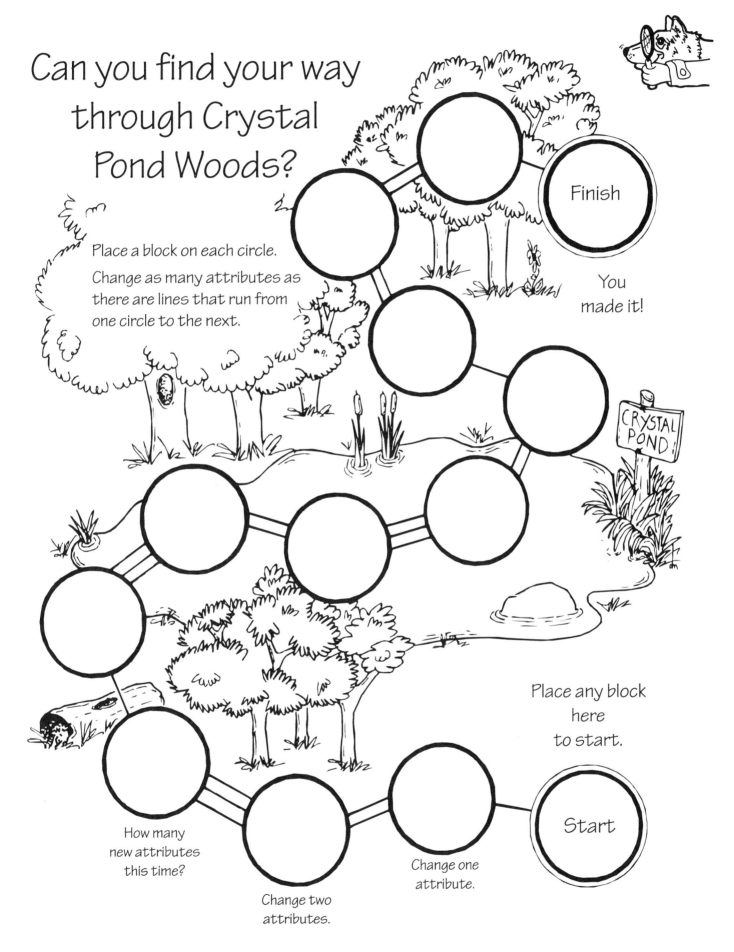

Place a block on each circle.

Change as many attributes as there are lines that run from one circle to the next.

Finish

You made it!

CRYSTAL POND

Place any block here to start.

Start

Change one attribute.

How many new attributes this time?

Change two attributes.

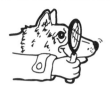

DETECTIVE THINKING
SMALL GROUP
LESSON 2

PURPOSE

The purpose of this lesson is to allow students to practice deductive thinking through the use of **Venn diagrams**. The teacher will give guided practice using Venn diagrams, followed by students working independently to demonstrate understanding.

TEACHER MATERIALS

— one copy of *The Birthday Present* story
— a class display of the dots that accompany *The Birthday Present*
— a set of markers   — a duplicated class set of *Friendly Clues*
— a duplicated class set of *Dudley's Dog Bones*

STUDENT MATERIALS

— pencil   — scissors

LESSON PLAN

1. Introduce students to the concept of *Venn Diagrams* by reading the story *The Birthday Present.* As the story is being read, the teacher will lead students through the process of using a Venn Diagram. The teacher may choose to have the dots drawn on chart paper or an overhead transparency and add the corresponding loops as described in the story. An alternative is to provide students with a duplicated copy of the dots to add the corresponding loops themselves. Be careful to loop the dots as described so the story will work.

2. Give students a copy of *Friendly Clues*. After reading the animal labels at the bottom of the page, have students cut them out and place them in the correct sections of Venn View 1. Labels from the intersection of Venn View 1 are then used to complete Venn View 2. Other labels are discarded. *(Answer: frog)*

3. Give students a copy of *Dudley's Dog Bones.* Have students cut out the numbered trees and place them correctly in the Venn Views using the same process as in *Friendly Clues. (Answer: 15)*

DIAGNOSTIC NOTES

Look for students who demonstrate a quick grasp of the concept of Venn diagrams by recognizing that each animal or number has only one correct space on the diagram. Students who correctly see the overlapping attributes also show strong potential. Some students may also be able to leap intuitively to correct responses without working the entire diagram.

The Birthday Present

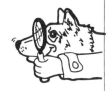

Dudley the Detective loves to play games with his friends in Crystal Pond Woods. In fact, he loves them so much that he often makes up games to challenge his friends with mysteries. On a bright, clear Saturday morning, Dudley was going to a birthday party Sybil the Scientist was giving for Felix Frog. Many of Dudley's best friends would be there, including Rascal Raccoon, Yolanda the Yarnspinner, Rosalyn Robin, Isabel the Inventor, Max the Magician, and many other creatures from Crystal Pond Woods. Dudley was especially excited about going to this party, because he was very proud of the game he had created for Felix Frog and his other friends to play during the celebration.

When Dudley reached Sybil's house, the party was just getting started. The friends played many party games, including "Hide the Acorn" and "Pin the Tail on the Tadpole." (Dudley secretly thought his game would be the most fun of all.) The friends ate cake, and then it was time for Felix Frog to open his presents. When the pile of presents was gone, Rosalyn Robin turned to Dudley. "You didn't bring a present for Felix!" she scolded.

"Oh, yes, I did," Dudley replied. "I drew Felix a picture of himself."

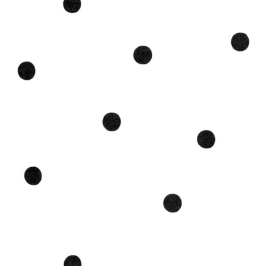

"Oh boy, let me see it!" Felix exclaimed excitedly.

Dudley held out his picture for all to see. Felix Frog looked disappointed. "I don't see myself," he said sadly. "It just looks like a bunch of black dots."

"That's because we have to play a game to find out which dot is you," Dudley replied.

Tommy Turtle squealed happily. "Is it a detective game?" he asked excitedly.

"Yes," smiled Dudley,"it is." He drew an orange ring around some of the dots on his picture.

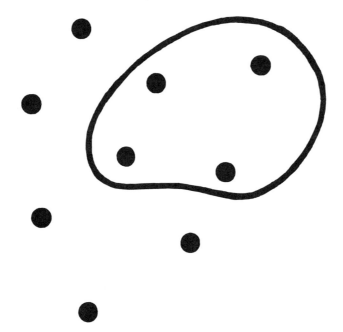

"The dots inside the orange ring are all of us who hop along the ground," said Dudley.

"Oh," sighed Tommy. "Then I am not in your ring. With my heavy shell and short legs, I certainly do not hop."

"That's all right," said Yolanda. "Even with all my eight legs, I cannot hop. So my dot would not be in the ring either."

Rosalyn chirped happily. "I would be in the orange ring, because when I am not flying in the air, I hop along the ground to look for tasty worms and bugs. But Max, Sybil and Felix would be in the orange ring, too, so I still do not know which dot is for me."

Dudley then drew a purple ring on the drawing. "Everyone inside the purple ring lays eggs," he said. "That is your second clue."

"Then I am outside of both rings," said Rascal. "I do not hop or lay eggs. But then, neither do you, Dudley, nor does Isabel."

"I do not lay eggs, and neither does Sybil," said Max. "But both kangaroos and rabbits hop, so these two dots must be for us."

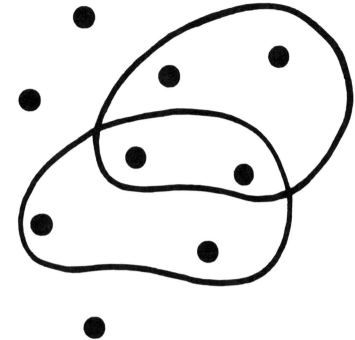

"That is correct. But what would Felix, the birthday guest of honor, be?" Dudley asked in a mysterious voice.

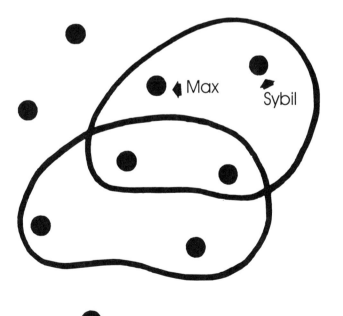

"Well," said Felix, "I hop along the ground, _and_ frogs lay eggs. So I must be one of these dots in the purple ring and the orange ring, too."

"Very good," Dudley agreed.

"I would be in the purple ring," said Tommy. "Turtles lay eggs. Yolanda, you would be in the purple ring, too. But which of the dots is mine?"

Dudley smiled a mysterious smile and drew a green ring on his picture.

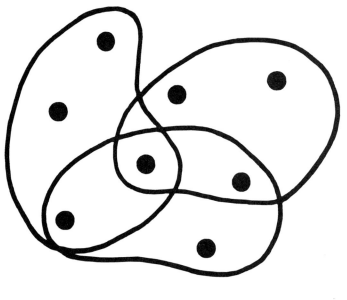

"Now for your third clue," he said. "Everyone in the green ring hibernates through the winter."

"That certainly leaves me out," said Yolanda. "Spiders most certainly do not hibernate."

"Then I know which dot is you!" cried Tommy. "You are the dot who lays eggs, but does not hop or hibernate! I know which dot is me, too, and which dot is Rosalyn!"

CAN YOU FIND ROSALYN'S DOT AND TOMMY'S DOT?

Isabel cried out excitedly, "I know where my dot goes, too! My cousins, the tree squirrels, do not hibernate through the winter, but we ground squirrels do, so my dot would be here, with Rascal Raccoon."

I know which dot is me, too!" shouted Felix happily. "I can even tell which dot belongs to you, Dudley! This was the best gift of all!" Felix cried. "Now I see that this IS a picture of me, and of you, too. This is a picture of my entire birthday party!"

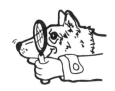

The Birthday Present
The Answer

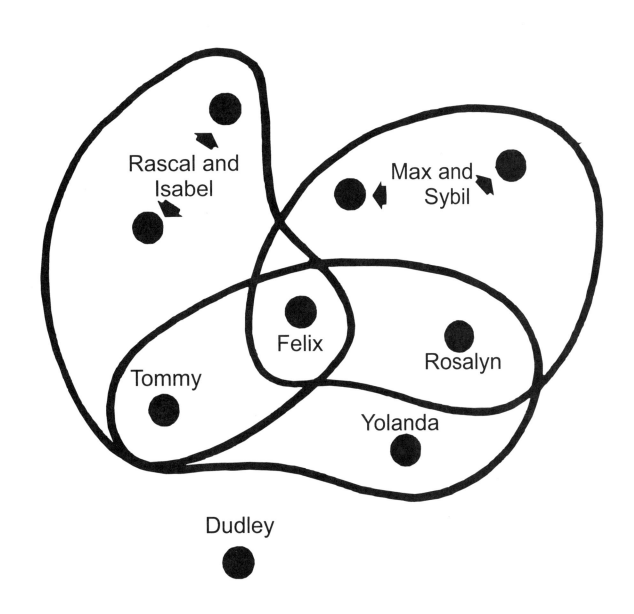

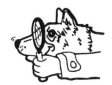

The Birthday Present

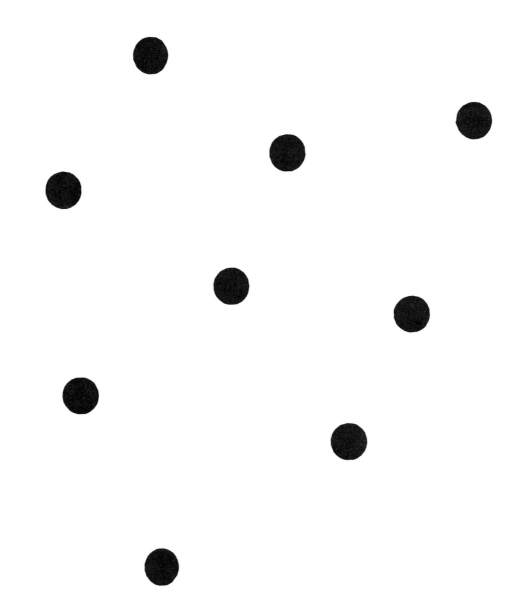

Can you find Felix's dot? Which belongs to Dudley?

Name _____

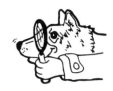

Friendly Clues

Dudley the Detective is having some forest friends join him for his birthday party. One of his friends is bringing a surprise guest.

Cut out the animal words. Use the clues to fit them into the correct sections of Venn View 1. Then move the names from the center of Venn View 1 into the correct sections of Venn View 2. Who is Dudley's surprise guest?

Venn View 1

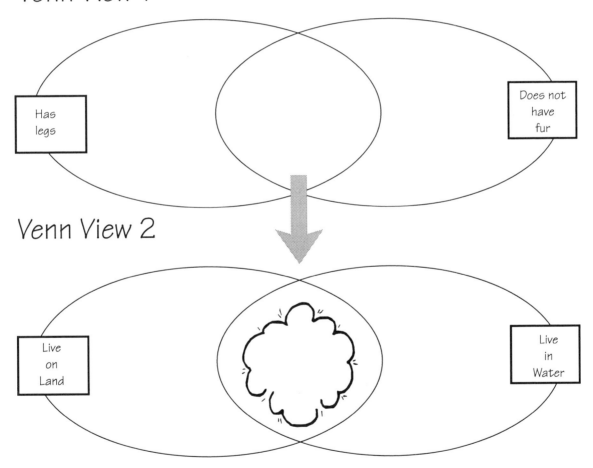

bear	lizard	bee	eagle	fish	snake	squirrei
spider	rabbit	raccoon	frog	robin	fox	crayfish

Dudley's Dog Bones

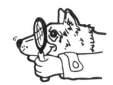

Dudley the Detective often buries his bones beneath the trees in Crystal Pond Woods. So he will not forget where he's hidden them, Dudley has numbered each tree in the woods. He has also drawn special Venn Views of Crystal Pond Woods that include clues to help him remember.

Cut out the trees and fit them into the Venn Views using Dudley's clues. Under which numbered tree will Dudley's dog bones be found?

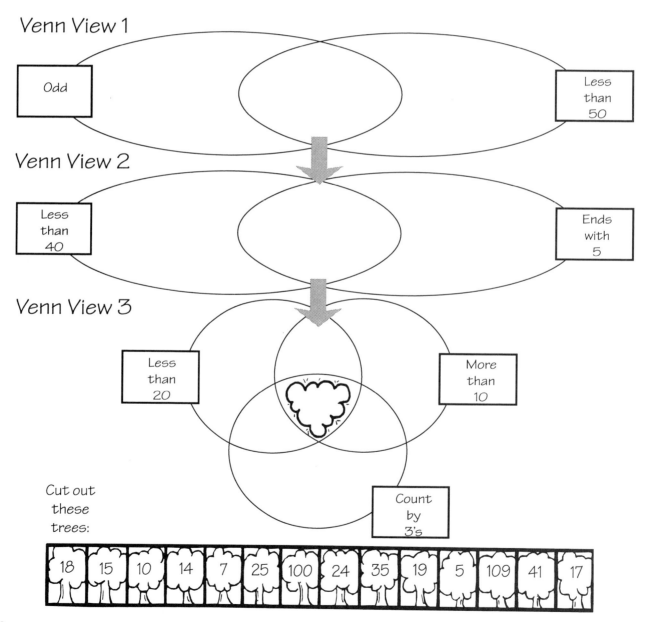

Venn View 1

Odd

Less than 50

Venn View 2

Less than 40

Ends with 5

Venn View 3

Less than 20

More than 10

Count by 3's

Cut out these trees:

| 18 | 15 | 10 | 14 | 7 | 25 | 100 | 24 | 35 | 19 | 5 | 109 | 41 | 17 |

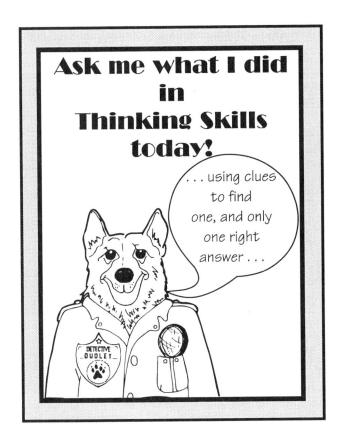

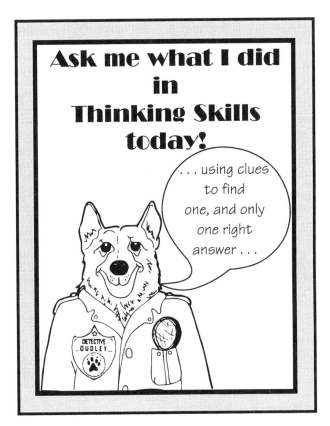

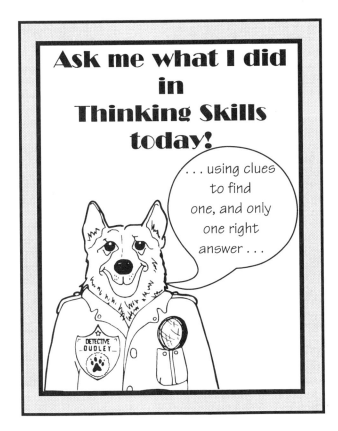

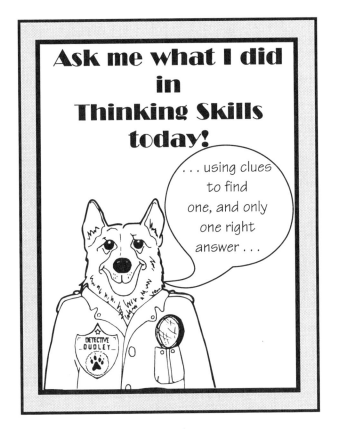

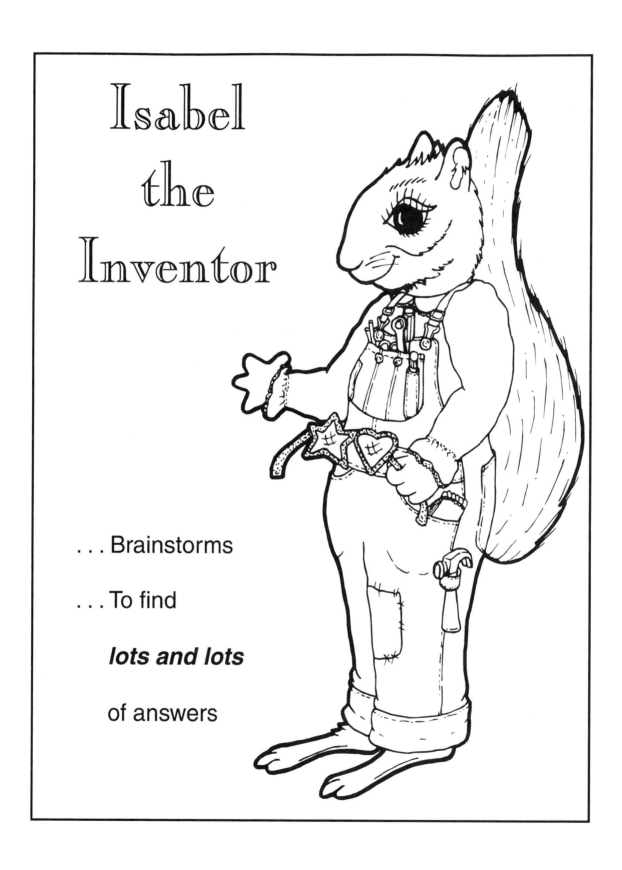

Isabel the Inventor

. . . Brainstorms

. . . To find

lots and lots

of answers

Isabel
the
Inventor

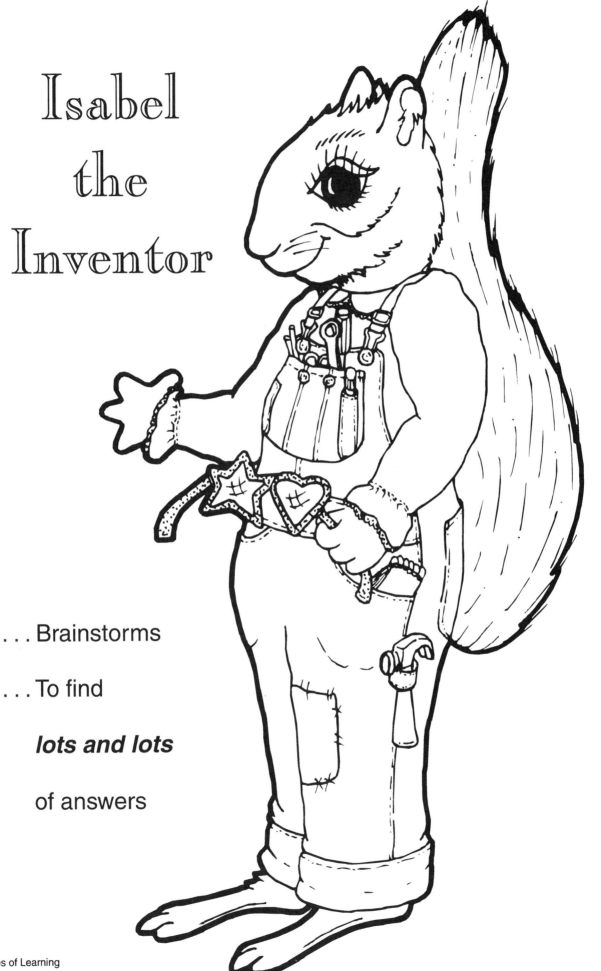

. . . Brainstorms

. . . To find

lots and lots

of answers

Divergent / Inventive Thinking

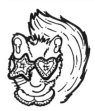

INVENTOR THINKING
WHOLE CLASS
LESSON 1

PURPOSE

The purpose of this lesson is to introduce students to **divergent production**. The students will be introduced to *Isabel the Inventor* who is able to see extraordinary possibilities in ordinary, everyday items. The lesson introduces the following concepts:
— There are many correct responses.
— It is important to see things creatively.
— It is encouraged to piggyback ideas from those of others.

TEACHER MATERIALS

— one copy of the *Isabel the Inventor* story to read aloud to the students
— a whisk (another kitchen utensil may be substituted)
— an overhead transparency of the picture of *Isabel the Inventor* and/or a class set of duplicated pictures for the students to color
— a duplicated class set of *BRAINFOCALS*™
— a duplicated class set of *Bubble Bonanza*
— a duplicated class set of *Yolanda's Cycle*
— Behavioral Checklist - *Inventor Thinking*

STUDENT MATERIALS

— crayons or markers
— pencils
— scissors
— glue

LESSON PLAN

1. Introduce the lesson by asking students if they know what an *inventor* is. Brainstorm some inventors and their inventions. Be sure to include female inventors. Discuss with students what they think are some of the most important inventions. Point out to students that there is a difference between inventing something and discovering something. Students may try to suggest that Ben Franklin invented electricity. Franklin *discovered* electricity but did not *invent* it. A generator to produce electricity is an example of an invention. A discovery is something that already exists. An invention is a new idea or creation thought up by someone. The inventor is the first person to

conceive the idea. The inventor may not actually make the object. Sometimes an inventor will hire someone else to make it.

2. Tell the students that today they are going to meet *Isabel the Inventor* who thinks in a way that is different from her friends in Crystal Pond Woods. Using the overhead projector, show students the picture of Isabel (page 50). You may wish to have them color the picture of Isabel (page 51) at this time or following the reading of the story.

3. Read the story and introduce Isabel the Inventor. At the appropriate points in the story encourage students to think about changing the size of the whisk, imagining it to be larger or smaller. Teachers do not have to use a whisk; any type of utensil will work.

4. Review with students these points from the story:

— In divergent thinking, there are many correct responses.
— It is important to be able to see ordinary things in new and unusual ways.
— Unusual and wacky ideas are to be encouraged.
— It is OK (and should be encouraged) to piggyback ideas.

5. Ask students if they would like special *Brainfocals™* to help them see things in new and different ways. Help students cut out and try on the *Brainfocals™, the memory trigger for this unit. Copying the master for the Brainfocals™* on brightly colored construction paper will provide students with the opportunity to mix and match colors. Students have the option of using the same shape and color or using different shapes and colors. Teachers may want to cut out the *Brainfocal™* pieces ahead of time.

6. Introduce *Bubble Bonanza* by having students put on their *Brainfocals ™* and look at the bubbles. Ask students to think about all of the possible things the bubbles could be. Ask students to draw what they see when they look at the bubbles. Teachers should collect *Bubble Bonanza* when students are finished and score them. Suggestions for assessing student work are provided in **DIAGNOSTIC NOTES.**

CHALLENGE PAGE

Yolanda's Cycle

DIAGNOSTIC NOTES

During the whole class lesson, the teacher and observer are looking for students who have many unusual and creative ideas. Students who display much enthusiasm during the activity should be observed carefully. In addition to many ideas, also look for students who will elaborate on their ideas.

A checklist for the whole class lessons is provided. The following is a short summary of what to look for in student behaviors.

LISTS MANY RESPONSES - All responses are acceptable. Look for students who provide many.

ELABORATES - This behavior would be displayed by a student who spends a long time adding details that other students would not think of. A student who piggybacks ideas of other students would be noted here.

SENSE OF HUMOR - Many talented students have an advanced sense of humor. The divergent thinking activities provide opportunities for students to display this sense of humor.

OFF-BEAT, ORIGINAL RESPONSES - Record the students with ideas that are very different. The ideas may be so wacky that they could not actually be implemented but the originality should be noted on the checklist.

ABILITY TO CHANGE COURSE - This reflects a student's flexibility of thought. Note the students that are truly able to see items in a variety of new ways.

ADVANCED VOCABULARY - These are the students who correctly use words classmates do not know. They sound very adult in the way in which they express themselves.

Bubble Bonanza

To score the student work, award one point for each completed picture. If two or more bubbles are combined into one drawing, score one point for each bubble involved. Award one point for each idea found only on that worksheet. Ideas that are similar yet different in at least one concept may be counted for both students. Award one point for each bubble that includes minute detail.

Yolanda's Cycle

Look for students who display a creative or elaborate design. In order to use this challenge page as a diagnostic tool, students must have the opportunity to work on it independently and in class.

NOTES

PETS

Behavioral Checklist

Inventor Thinking
(Inventive Thinking/Divergent)

List names of students as each behavior appears.
  Add checkmarks after name if behavior is repeated.
  Use a different color of ink or pencil for each whole group lesson.

Teacher _____
Grade: 1 ___ 2 ___ 3 ___

Dates of whole   1. _____
group instruction: 2. _____

LISTS MANY RESPONSES (fluency)	*OFFERS OFF-BEAT* AND/OR *ORIGINAL IDEAS* (originality)
EASILY *ELABORATES* OR *EXPANDS ON AN IDEA* (elaboration)	CHANGES COURSE -- *STARTS NEW CATEGORIES* OF RESPONSES (flexibility)
DISPLAYS AN UNUSUAL/MATURE *SENSE OF HUMOR*	*ADVANCED VOCABULARY* -- CAN EXPRESS SELF IN A MATURE, ARTICULATE MANNER
PETS classwork indicates an outstanding ability to use this thinking skill.	The following student/s did not participate during the thinking skills lessons, but I see these behaviors during **regular class time**.

ISABEL THE INVENTOR

One day as Yolanda the Yarnspinner was cleaning house she discovered an object she had never seen before and did not know what it was. (*Show the class a whisk.)*

She knew that if she wanted to find out the correct name for the object, Dudley the Detective was the person to ask. She hopped on her bicycle and rode off to Dudley's house. Dudley knew the object immediately.

"Yolanda," said Dudley, "this is a whisk. It is used in the kitchen to mix ingredients such as eggs."

Yolanda was very impressed. Because she never cooks, she did not have a need for a whisk. Yet it was such an interesting object that she did not want to give it away. What could she do with it? Of course that would require visiting another friend of Yolanda's, Isabel the Inventor, who lived in a tree in Crystal Pond Woods.

Isabel the Inventor is a very special person in Crystal Pond Woods. She loves to think but in a different way than Dudley. Isabel likes to think about things in **new and different ways**. She loves to invent new things and different ways of doing things.

Isabel has very special glasses that help her see things in a different way. Her glasses are similar to bifocals but are called Brainfocals™ When Isabel puts on her Brainfocals™, her brain begins **brainstorming ideas**. She is then able to see unusual possibilities in everyday things. When her ideas begin to flow, there is no stopping her.

Yolanda knocked on the door and entered Isabel's storage room. It was full of many wonderful, interesting items including a huge pile of nuts. Isabel's favorite saying was "I like to store as many nutty ideas as I do nuts."

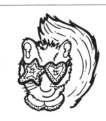

"Isabel," said Yolanda, "I found this in my house today, and Dudley told me it is a whisk. You know that I never cook so I never have any ingredients to mix. I hate to throw it away because it looks so interesting. Can you help me figure out what to do with it?"

Isabel loves challenges and was excited to have a chance to do some brainstorming. "Of course, I would love to brainstorm some ideas with you."

Isabel began to look at the whisk from all different angles. She considered a number of possibilities, like a drumstick or a rug beater, but none of them seemed very interesting.

"Wait, Yolanda!" Isabel exclaimed. "I need my Brainfocals™! You've heard of **bi**focals that help people see, right? Well, Brainfocals™ help focus my brain so I see things in new and different ways!" Isabel excitedly put on her Brainfocals™.

Her eyes behind her Brainfocals™ began to sparkle. "Wow, now I can think of many ways to use this! It could be a tree ornament . . . or a hanging plant holder . . . or a hair curler."

Yolanda could tell that Isabel was having a great time coming up with ideas. She wanted to try, too. Isabel helped Yolanda make a pair of Brainfocals™ so she could also see the whisk in more new and different ways. Yolanda began to add ideas to the list. Isabel and Yolanda were getting some very unusual ideas.

(At this point, brainstorm with students other possible uses for the whisk. Encourage unusual ideas, but accept all ideas. Include the idea of using the whisk as a bubble blower.)

Finally Isabel and Yolanda had filled up the paper with ideas.

"Wow, Isabel," exclaimed Yolanda, "you are right about storing many nutty ideas. I loved all of your ideas, but my favorite idea is to use the whisk to blow bubbles. I need to find some bubble-blowing solution."

"Don't worry," said Isabel, "I don't have any bubble-blowing solution, but I'll bet we can invent our own. Then we can go outside and spend the afternoon blowing bubbles."

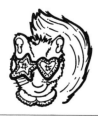

Brainfocals™

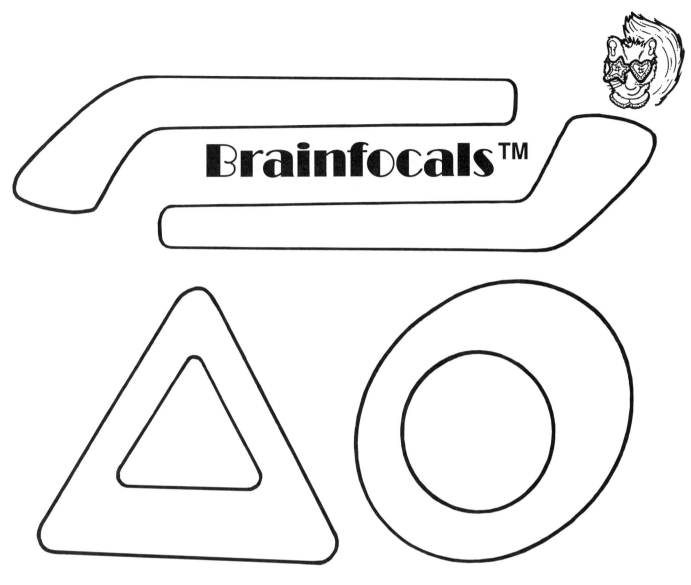

Cut out the 2 arms and any 2 shapes.
Glue together and decorate.

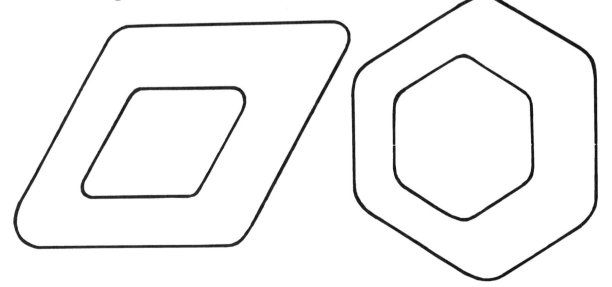

Bubble Bonanza

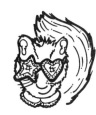

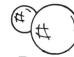
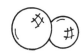

Using your Brainfocals,™ look at Isabel's bubbles in new and different ways. Draw what you "see."

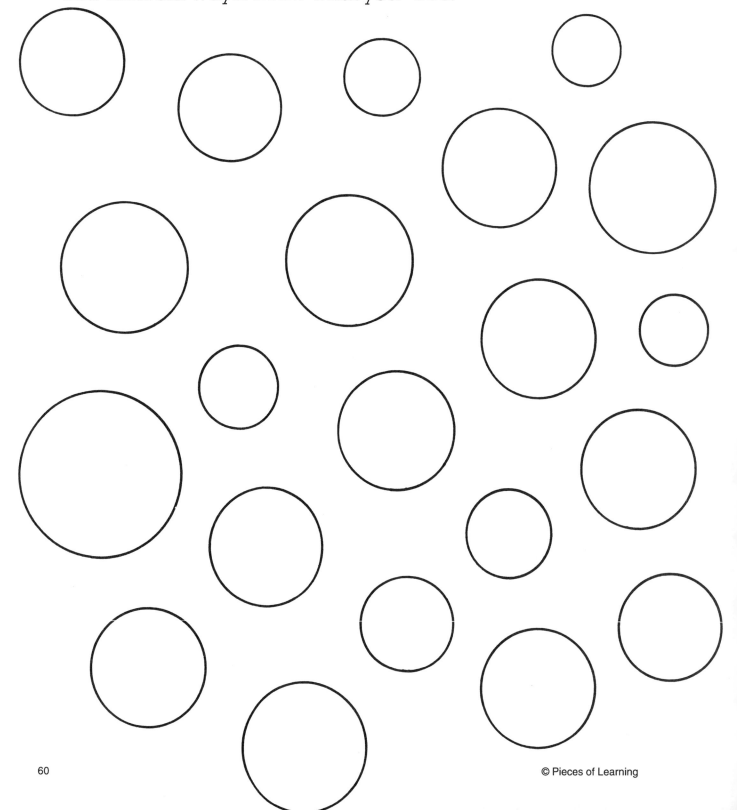

Name _____

Yolanda's Cycle

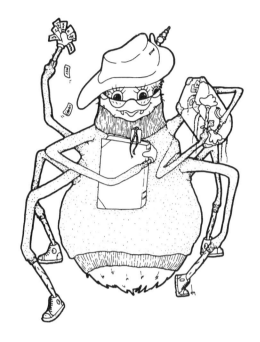

Your <u>bi</u>cycle has 2 wheels and 2 pedals. Help Isabel the Inventor design a new **spicycle** for her friend, Yolanda. Remember — Yolanda's a spider and has 8 legs!

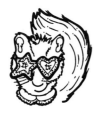

INVENTOR THINKING
WHOLE CLASS
LESSON 2

PURPOSE

The purpose of this lesson is to review and develop **divergent production of ideas**. The lesson extends and supports the concepts covered in Lesson 1.

TEACHER MATERIALS

— one duplicated classroom set of *Help Me, Help Me* and *Some Spare Parts*
— one duplicated classroom set of *The Great Acorn Collection and Storage Machine*
— Behavioral Checklist - *Inventor Thinking*

STUDENT MATERIALS

— crayons or markers
— pencils
— scissors
— glue
— tape

LESSON PLAN

1. Review the characteristics of inventive thinking.
   — In divergent thinking, there are many correct responses.
   — It is important to be able to see ordinary things in new and unusual ways.
   — Unusual and wacky ideas are to be encouraged.
   — It is OK to piggyback ideas.

2. Discuss with students that many times inventors are also *problem solvers.* An example of this is in the first automobiles that were designed and driven. The drivers were unable to see while it was raining so someone fixed the problem by inventing windshield wipers. Brainstorm with students other inventions that were the result of a problem that needed to be solved.

3. Introduce the activity by explaining to students that Sybil needs to get across the pond. Brainstorm with students ways she might get across the pond. Possibilities might

include floating, flying, or going underwater. Explain that Isabel has a variety of things or spare parts she can use in creating or building something to cross the pond. Give students *Help Me, Help Me* and *Some Spare Parts*. The students' task is to design or create something to help Sybil cross the pond. Students need to use at least two of the spare parts. They may use more and may include items or ideas of their own. Some of the spare parts will not look familiar to students. Encourage students to think of uses for the part despite the fact they may not know what it is.

4. After students have completed the worksheets, collect them for further assessment.

CHALLENGE PAGE

The Great Acorn Collection and Storage Machine

5. The Challenge Page provides students with additional opportunities for creating and designing new things. The two worksheets need to be copied on separate sheets of paper and taped together. The two sheets will provide students with ample space for their designs.

DIAGNOSTIC NOTES

This lesson provides additional opportunities for students to display the same characteristics emphasized in Lesson 1. The following is a short summary of what to look for in student behaviors.

LISTS MANY RESPONSES - All responses are acceptable. Some students may cut out pieces to make a bridge across the pond. This is not creative and would not work unless all the pieces floated. Although all responses are acceptable, look for students who are willing to design a number of possibilities or design something more creative than a bridge.

ELABORATES - This behavior would be displayed by a student who spends a long time adding details that other students would not think of. Look for such detail.

SENSE OF HUMOR - Many talented students have an advanced sense of humor. The divergent thinking activities provide opportunities for students to display this sense of humor.

OFF-BEAT, ORIGINAL RESPONSES - Record the students with ideas that are very different. The ideas may be so wacky that they could not actually be implemented but the originality should be noted on the checklist. An example might be the student who uses the parts to build something three dimensional. Also look for students who add very creative parts of their own.

ABILITY TO CHANGE COURSE - This reflects a student's flexibility of thought. Note the students that are truly able to see items in a variety of new ways. They may use one of the spare parts in a way not usually intended.

ADVANCED VOCABULARY - These are the students who correctly use words classmates do not know. They sound very adult in the way in which they express themselves.

The Great Acorn Collection and Storage Machine
When assessing *The Great Acorn Collection and Storage Machine* look for the same type of behaviors noted for the Whole Class Lesson. Elaboration and original ideas are the most easily assessed concepts.

NOTES

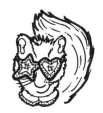

"Help Me! Help Me!"

Sybil the Scientist needs something that will help her get across Crystal Pond. Create an invention to help her out — use at least two of Isabel the Inventor's spare parts that are on the next page.

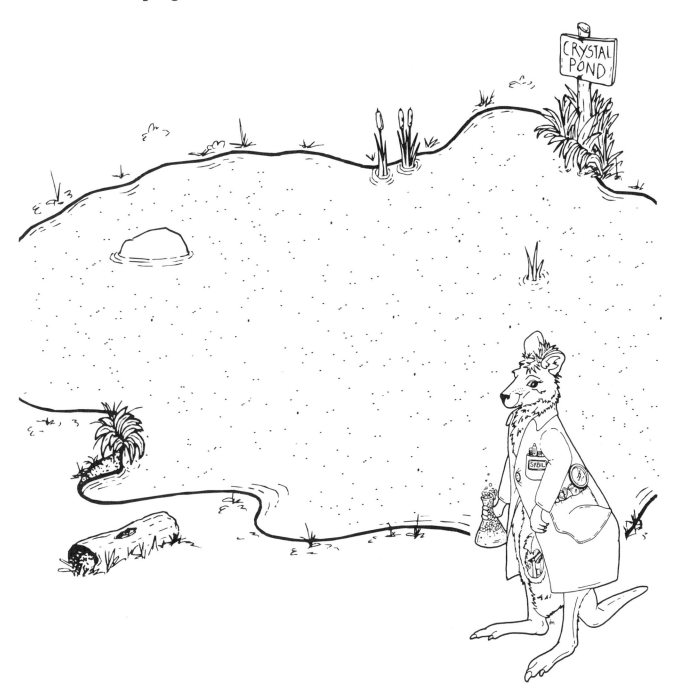

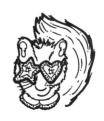

Here are a few spare parts from Isabel the Inventor's workshop. Use at least 2 of these parts to help get Sybil the Scientist across Crystal Pond.

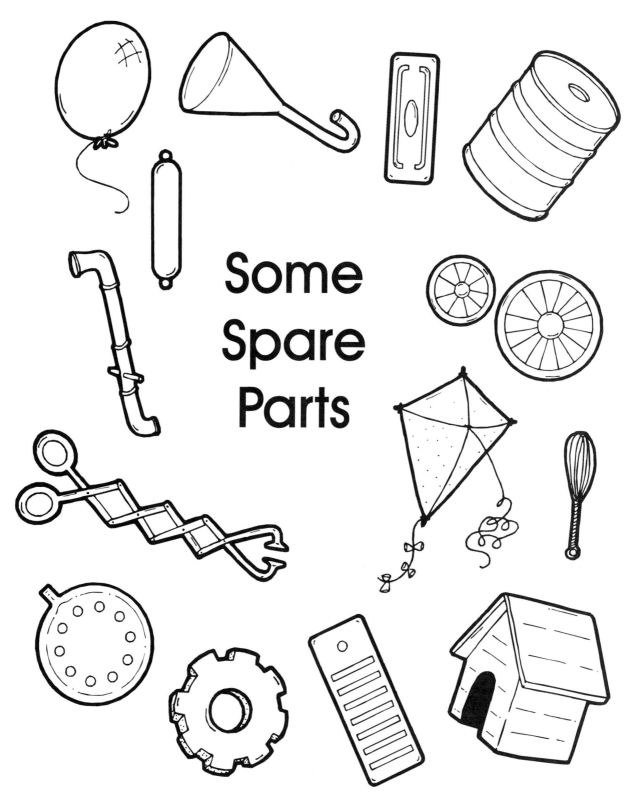

Some Spare Parts

Name _____

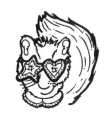

Winter is coming. The acorns that Isabel eats during the long winter months are still scattered on the ground all over Crystal Pond Woods. She needs your help! Invent a machine to gather acorns and take them to Isabel's hollow near the top of this big tree. Draw and label your invention.

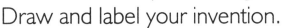

The Great Acorn Collection and Storage Machine

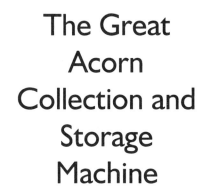

ISABEL

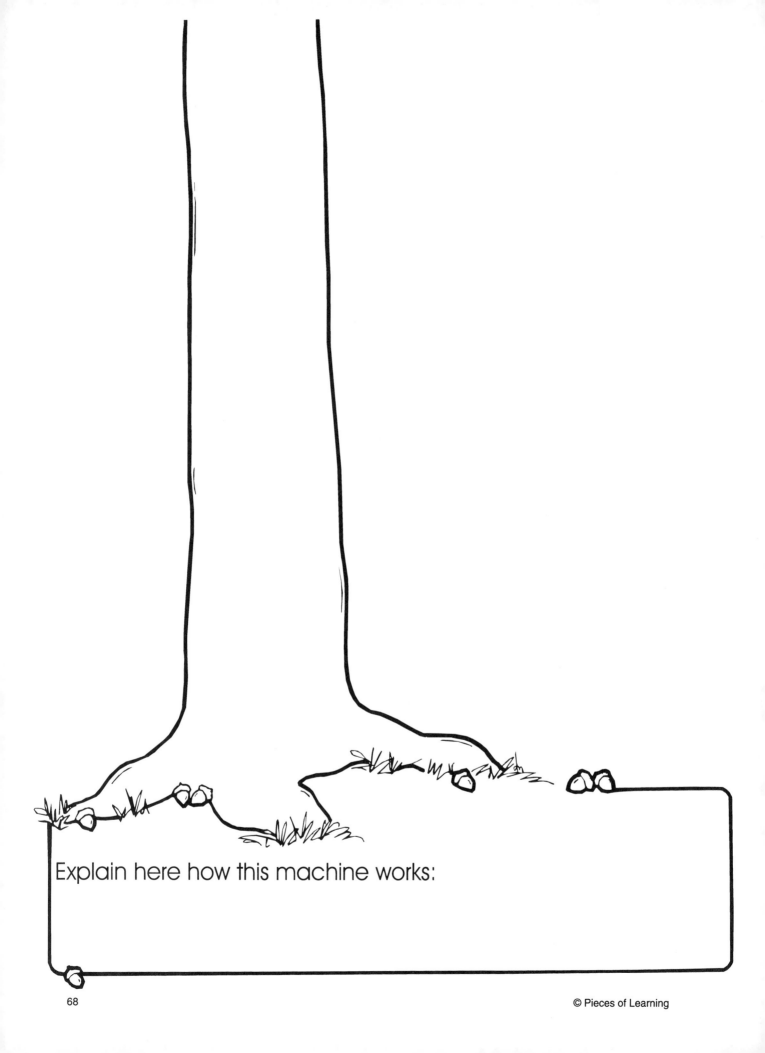

Explain here how this machine works:

INVENTOR THINKING
SMALL GROUP
LESSON 1

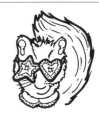

PURPOSE

The purpose of this lesson is to give students the opportunity to display their **creative thinking.** Based on the research of Dr. E. Paul Torrance, the creative thinker is defined as one who has many ideas (fluency), in many different categories (flexibility), is original (originality), and shows detail (elaboration). The lesson will provide another outlet for the creative thinker.

TEACHER MATERIALS

— a duplicated class set of *Unique Ideas*

STUDENT MATERIALS

— crayons or markers
— pencil

LESSON PLAN

1. The following is a short story lead-in to the activity. It can be read to students or the directions can be given verbally.

Isabel found these parts of pictures hidden in the bottom of the big oak tree near Rascal Raccoon's home. She thought the pictures were very interesting, but they are not finished. After putting on her Brainfocals™, she saw many possibilities for finishing the pictures.

Directions: *Use your imagination to finish the pictures. Imagine what the pictures could be. Then add color and lines to finish them.*

2. Because elaboration (adding details) takes time, it is important to give students plenty of time. To ensure individual creativity, students should not sit next to each other. Do not offer advice to students. It is creative if students join pictures and draw outside the boxes. It would not necessarily be creative if the teacher suggests this.

3. It may be necessary to ask students to describe their pictures and for the teacher to caption the pictures. This will help during the assessment of creativity.

DIAGNOSTIC NOTES

This activity can be numerically scored to assess student creativity. Points are awarded based on fluency, flexibility, originality and elaboration. To score the student pictures, use tally marks on the scoring grid at the bottom of the *Unique Ideas* worksheet. Combine the tally marks for a total creativity score.

Scoring for fluency: Award one point for each completed picture. If two or more squares are combined into one drawing, score one point for each square involved.

Scoring for flexibility: Award one point for each new category depicted. *(An example would be when a student draws an animal, then an outer space picture, and then a landscape.)*

Scoring for originality: Scan all worksheets from the group. Award one point for each idea found only on that worksheet. *(An example would be the student who made the top right picture into a piano keyboard when no one else did.)* Ideas that are similar yet different in at least one concept may be counted for both students. Combining squares takes extra creativity and daring. Award a point for each combined squares picture.

Scoring for elaboration: Award one point for each square in which lines or shapes that are significant to the picture have been drawn outside of the box. This does not include combined squares which have already been evaluated. Award one point for each drawing that includes minute detail.

NOTES

Name _____

Unique Ideas

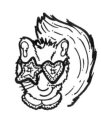

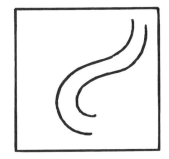 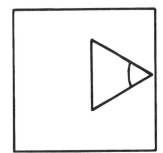 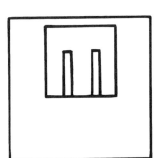

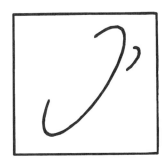 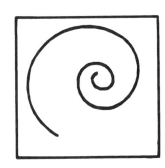 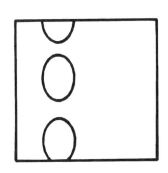

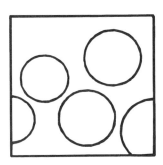 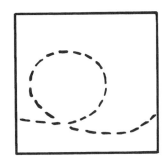 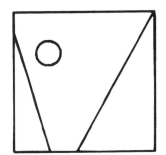

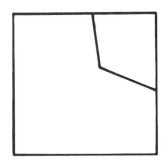 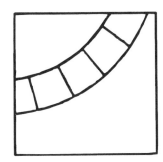 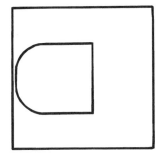

F	O
F	E

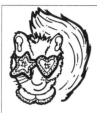

INVENTOR THINKING
SMALL GROUP
LESSON 2

PURPOSE

The purpose of the lesson is to allow students to practice their **inventive thinking** by **combining** shapes with locations to think up many possibilities. In the small group setting and game situation, students who are not as vocal as their classmates have to participate. The teacher should encourage fluency, flexibility, and originality.

TEACHER MATERIALS

— one copy of the game board *WHAT MIGHT THIS BE?*
— colored game pieces or game markers to move around the board
— beans or counters for keeping score
— a die
— the spinner for *WHAT MIGHT THIS BE?*
— something which times one minute

STUDENT MATERIALS

— a colored game piece or game marker to move around the board

LESSON PLAN

1. Students are going to play the game *WHAT MIGHT THIS BE?* The four worksheets for the game board are provided and should be cut out and put together prior to the small group lesson. A copy of the spinner is also provided. A picture of how the completed game board should look is included. Students will need some type of game piece for moving around the board.

2. The instructions for *WHAT MIGHT THIS BE?* are as follows:

— Have students place their game piece on any square of the game board.

— On their turn, students roll the die and move the appropriate number of spaces around the board. On their first move, students select the direction their game piece will move; subsequent moves continue in the same direction.

— After moving their game piece, students spin the spinner.

— Students are given one minute to name all the items they can think of which fit the category indicated by combining the shape spun and the location shown on their square on the path. For example: If a student lands on a square marked "beside your bed" and spins an oval shape, the student tries to name as many things as possible which are oval shaped beside a bed.

3. Scoring the game is done by the teacher. Students receive one point for each item they name which fits the category. Teachers should be generous in scoring so as not to stifle creative thinking. Err on the side of generosity. The teacher may choose to award two points for answers that are highly creative or unique. Students take one counter for each point they receive on each round.

If students cannot think of a response on their turn in the one minute provided, they pay a counter back to the pot. The teacher may want to impose a penalty of paying one counter if students talk during another student's turn. This will ensure that quiet students have a chance to participate. The winner is the student with the most counters.

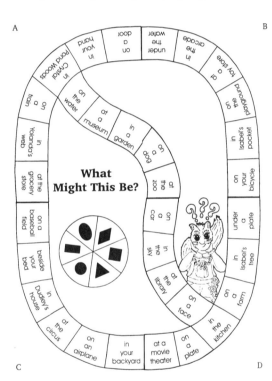

DIAGNOSTIC NOTES

As students play the game, listen for creative, unique responses. Watch for students who list a great many responses. Note students who can think flexibly, branching into new categories. Students who give original responses show special potential. Some examples of creative responses given by students are the following:

SPINNER	SPACE ON BOARD	RESPONSE
▮	on face	number one on a clock
▲	on a car	a car carrying home a Christmas tree
●	on the water	the reflection of the moon
●	in the sky	a Frisbee

A

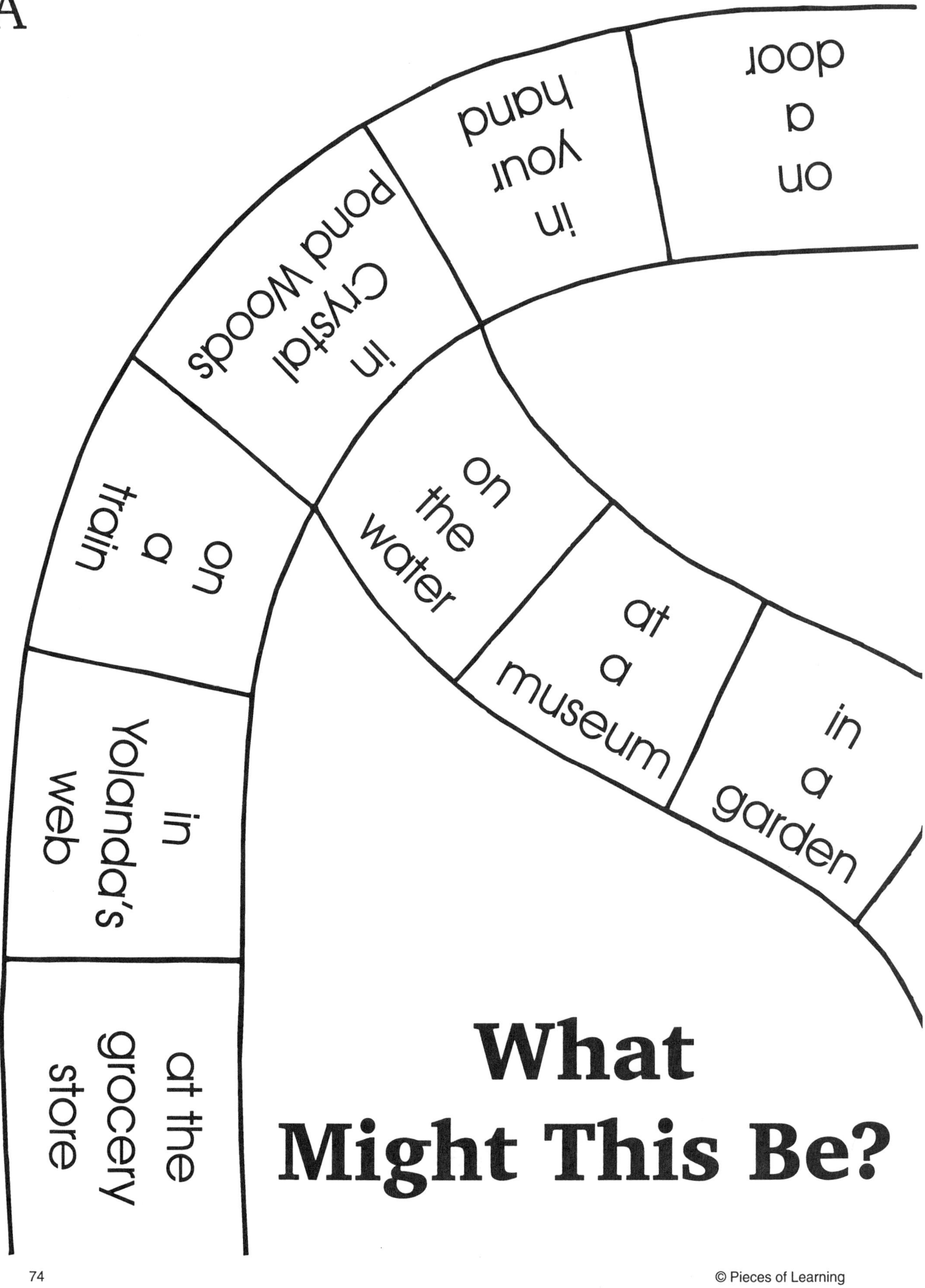

on
a door

in
your
hand

in
Crystal
pond Woods

on
a
train

on
the
water

at
a
museum

in
a
garden

in
Yolanda's
web

at the
grocery
store

What
Might This Be?

B

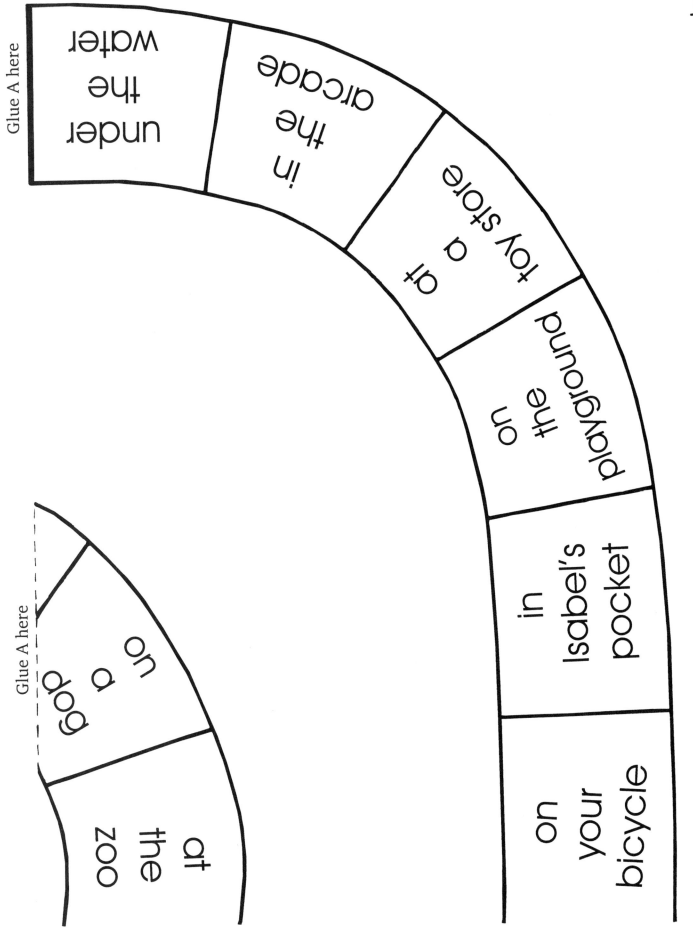

under the water

Glue A here

in the arcade

at a toy store

on the playground

in Isabel's pocket

on your bicycle

on a dog

at the zoo

Glue A here

Glue A here

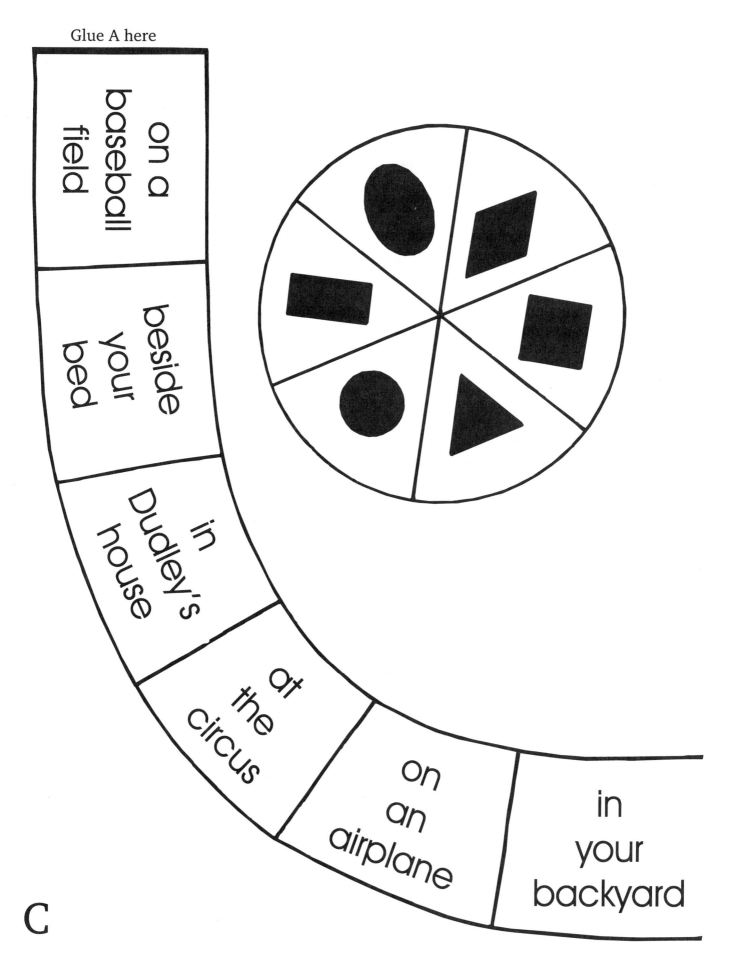

on a
baseball
field

beside
your
bed

in
Dudley's
house

at
the
circus

on
an
airplane

in
your
backyard

C

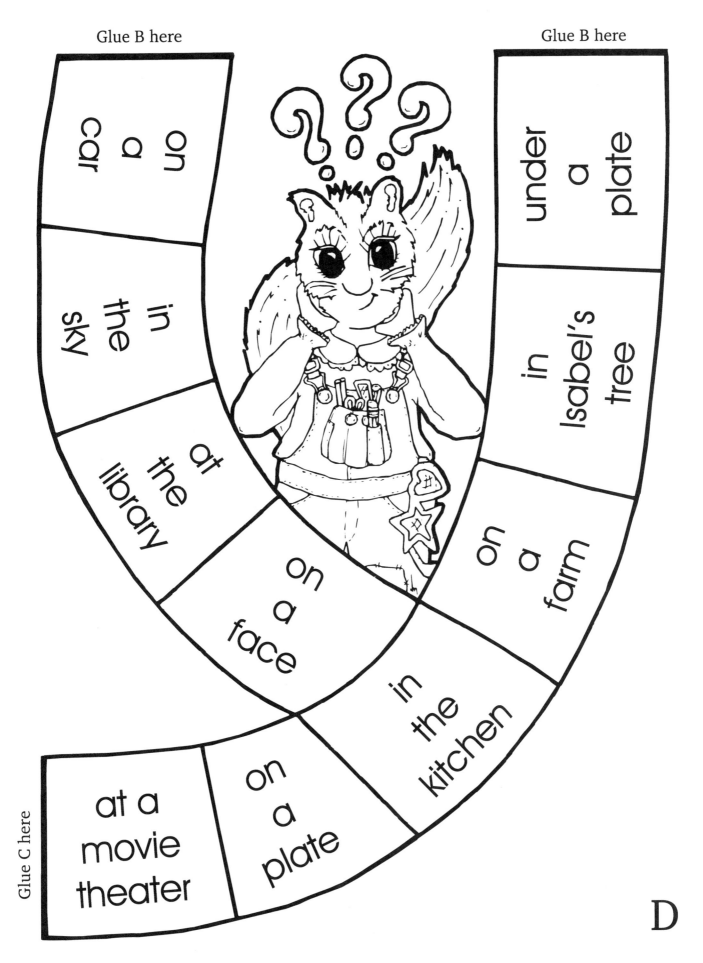

on
a
car

in
the
sky

at
the
library

on
a
face

under
a
plate

in
Isabel's
tree

on
a
farm

in
the
kitchen

on
a
plate

at a
movie
theater

D

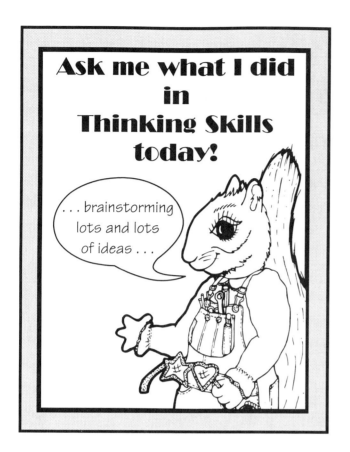

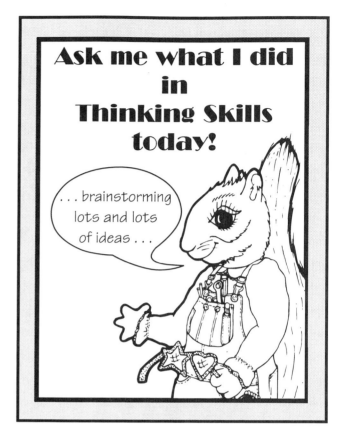

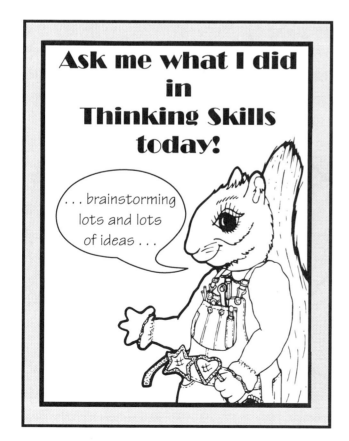

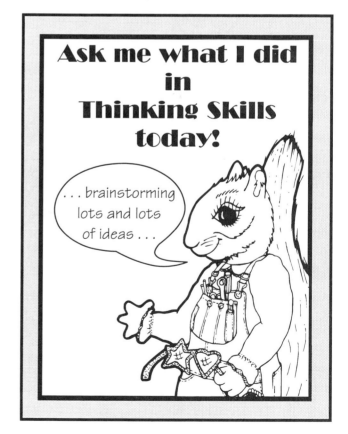

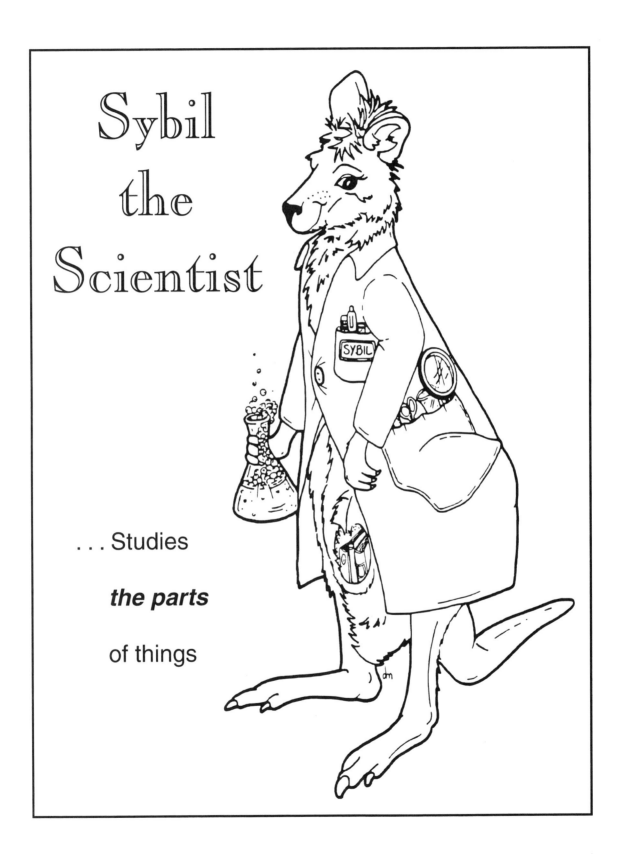

Sybil the Scientist

. . . Studies

the parts

of things

Sybil
the
Scientist

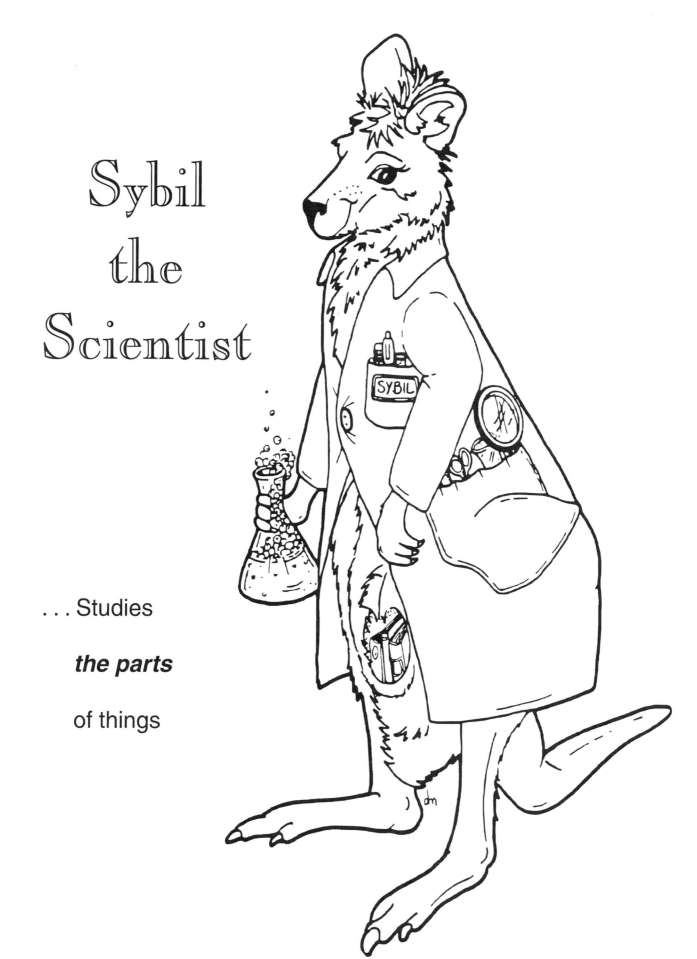

. . . Studies

the parts

of things

SCIENTIST THINKING
WHOLE CLASS
LESSON 1

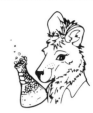

PURPOSE

The purpose of this lesson is to introduce the students to **analytical thinking**. They will meet Sybil, a scientist who loves to classify and organize the information she collects. The students will learn that in analytical thinking:

— There are no pre-determined rules for classifying. The scientist must classify data that has never been sorted and organized before, and it is up to her to determine the rules for sorting.
— There may be more than one equally correct way to sort data.

TEACHER MATERIALS

— one copy of the *Sybil the Scientist* story to read aloud to the students
— an overhead transparency of the picture of *Sybil the Scientist* and/or a class set of duplicated pictures for students to color
— a class set of magnifying glasses. Magnifying glasses can be purchased at a reasonable cost through catalogs such as *Oriental Trading Company* or through local dental offices. If magnifying glasses are not available, a duplicated class set of *Sybil's Magnifying Glass* will be needed.
— an overhead set of *Sybil's Creatures*. The overhead of *Sybil's Creatures* should be colored and cut out so they can be moved around easily. Use a variety of colors and color some creatures with two or more different colors.
— an overhead transparency of *Sybil's Laboratory*
— a duplicated class set of the *Loose Laboratory Limpets* and *Sybil's Laboratory*
— the Behavioral Checklist - *Scientist Thinking*

STUDENT MATERIALS

— pencils
— scissors
— glue

LESSON PLAN

1. Introduce the lesson by asking students if they know what a *scientist* does. Discuss scientists and any real life scientists known to students. Brainstorm the different kinds of things a scientist might study.

2. Introduce *Sybil the Scientist,* the new character, to students. Sybil is special because she thinks in a scientific way. Observations are very important to a scientist. Sybil uses all of her senses: tasting, seeing, hearing, smelling and touching. Many scientists use a magnifying glass. The magnifying glass allows more detailed observations of objects, especially small objects. During the story there is a place to point out the picture of Sybil and the fact that she is wearing a laboratory coat to protect her from spills. Sybil's laboratory coat has many pockets where she keeps her most important objects. During the reading of the story there is a place to discuss with students the items in her pockets. Sometimes, after a scientist has collected a lot of new data, it is important to organize or group the data. A fancy word for "group the data" is classify. Scientists read how other scientists classify because there are many ways to classify items.

3. Read the *Sybil the Scientist* story. During the story, students will be given actual magnifying glasses or a picture of a magnifying glass, the memory trigger for this unit. The whole class activity is part of the story. Toward the end of the story, students will pause to make some observations and classify the laboratory creatures. Use the overhead transparency of *Sybil's Laboratory* to classify the creatures. Remind students that the observations need to be as accurate as possible. When classifying the laboratory creatures into the four cages, it is important to accept any characteristic that makes sense. As students offer suggestions about how to classify the creatures, point out that the suggestions are called hypotheses, or educated guesses. It is normal for a scientist's hypothesis to change frequently. It is also quite possible that the class may not discover a workable hypothesis. That is part of science.

4. Review with students these points from the story:

   — When scientists receive new information, they put things into categories or groups that have common characteristics.
   — Scientists group the new information based on observations.
   — When categorizing new information, there are no rules. Hypotheses will change and evolve as they are tested.

CHALLENGE PAGES

Loose Laboratory Limpets
Sybil's Laboratory

5. Distribute the Challenge pages. When giving the directions to students for *Loose Laboratory Limpets* instruct students NOT to color the limpets. Decisions based on categorizing the limpets should take into account that the limpets are black and white.

Students should glue their limpets onto the *Sybil's Laboratory* worksheet. The following are some of the possible ways *Loose Laboratory Limpets* can be categorized:

1. dots	2. cow spots	3. stripes	4. 6 or more legs
1. smiling	2. open mouth	3. sad	4. straight/squiggly mouth
1. 3 legs	2. 4 legs	3. 2 or less legs	4. plain

DIAGNOSTIC NOTES

Look for students who are able to correctly sort the samples into discrete sets, so that each group has at least one item but no item fits equally well into more than one group. Students who are particularly capable of thinking analytically may be able to sort the data more than one way, each time applying one equally good set of classifiers.

A checklist for the whole class lesson is provided. The following is a short summary of what to look for in student behaviors.

IDENTIFIES ATTRIBUTES - Look for students who understand the concept of attributes. They understand that a creature that is blue and white cannot be categorized in the blue *and* in the white categories.

CREATES CLASSIFICATION SYSTEMS - Look for students who are able to create a classification system. Also look for the students who will try a sorting system that is unique. This system may not work, but the fact that they were willing to try something uniquely different is an important characteristic.

DEMONSTRATES UNIQUE STRATEGIES - Look for students who categorize or sort in an unusual or different way. These are the students who come up with ideas that few other students think of.

DEFERS JUDGMENT - Look for students who are able to change course and try new ideas. Some students will focus on one characteristic and not give up, even when it's obvious sorting by that characteristic will not work.

DRAWS RELATIONSHIPS BETWEEN LESSON AND OUTSIDE INFORMATION - Look for students who know or want to know specific facts about science. Some students will bring to class a vast knowledge about science topics. This in itself does not indicate a potentially talented student, but combined with some of the other characteristics will give the teacher a more complete picture of the student's potential.

RECOGNIZES FLAWED REASONING - Look for students who are able to recognize when a certain sorting system will not work.

Loose Laboratory Limpets and ***Sybil's Laboratory***
Look for students who are able to accurately sort all limpets into four discrete sets.

P E T S

Behavioral Checklist

Scientist Thinking

(Analysis/Convergent)

Teacher _____
Grade: 1 ___ 2 ___ 3 ___

Dates of whole   1. _____
group instruction: 2. _____

QUICKLY AND ACCURATELY *IDENTIFIES ATTRIBUTES*	CREATES *CLASSIFICATION SYSTEMS* THAT WORK
DEMONSTRATES UNIQUE STRATEGIES FOR ANALYZING	GATHERS AND WEIGHS ALL DATA BEFORE DECIDING ON AN ANSWER -- *DEFERS JUDGMENT*.
DRAWS RELATIONSHIPS BETWEEN LESSON AND OUTSIDE INFORMATION TO HELP DETERMINE CONCLUSIONS	*RECOGNIZES FLAWED REASONING*
PETS classwork indicates an outstanding ability to use this thinking skill.	The following student/s did not participate during the thinking skills lessons, but I see these behaviors during **regular class time**.

SYBIL THE SCIENTIST

It was a beautiful day in Crystal Pond Woods. The animals were outside enjoying the great weather and preparing for the annual Crystal Pond Picnic. All of the animals, that is, except for Sybil the Scientist.

A scientist is a very special person. One of the things a scientist does is make careful observations of the world around her. **Observation** is a fancy word for looking at things. But a scientist does not just look at things. Sybil uses all five senses: seeing, hearing, smelling, touching, and sometimes tasting. She carefully records this information, which she calls **data,** in her journal. As Sybil collects data or new information, she tries to **organize or categorize** the information according to **rules.**

Sybil wears a white laboratory coat to protect her from possible spills in the laboratory. Her laboratory coat has many pockets filled with her most important objects. One of the objects she always carries with her is a magnifying glass. The magnifying glass allows Sybil to observe objects more closely. What are some of the other objects Sybil carries? Can you think of some reasons why Sybil carries these items in her pockets?

(At this point engage the students in a discussion regarding the possible uses of the instruments. The books are especially important to scientists because they often read to learn more about the things that interest them. Scientists also read what other scientists are doing so they can compare data. The magnifying glass helps Sybil make more careful observations with her eyes. The scissors allow her to cut into things to see what they look like on the inside. The test tube allows Sybil to see what happens when she mixes things.

If using actual magnifying glasses, give them to students now. Students may need an opportunity to observe some items using

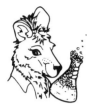

the magnifying glass. If actual magnifying glasses are not being used, give students a copy of Sybil's Magnifying Glass memory trigger to make. The purpose of the magnifying glass is to remind students how scientists think.)

Sybil works in a very exciting place — a laboratory. Sybil's laboratory is a very busy place with many experiments going on. Sybil is very curious and loves to make observations, set up experiments, and to think scientifically.

That day, as Sybil was writing her observations for the morning in her science journal, Jordan the Judge stopped by. Jordan and Sybil were going to play in the softball game at the annual picnic.

"Hi, Jordan," said Sybil. "I will be ready as soon as I finish recording my observations."

Sybil locked the laboratory, and they left to enjoy the softball game and Crystal Pond Woods picnic.

Sybil and Jordan never finished the softball game. Sybil chased a long fly ball into the woods and, while looking for the ball, she discovered a group of creatures she had never seen before! Sybil was very excited, as scientists are when they make a new discovery. Sybil, with Jordan's help, gathered the new creatures together and took them back to her laboratory where she could make careful observations.

Sybil was the first scientist in Crystal Pond Woods to discover the creatures. After she safely returned to her laboratory with the creatures, Sybil began to think scientifically. First, she read her science books to see if any other scientists had written about these creatures, but she could find no information in her books.

Next, she got a brand new science journal for her observations of the creatures. Sybil wanted to organize the new information about the creatures in order to classify them. **Classifying** is organizing into groups. Since no one had given her any rules to follow for creating her groups, Sybil had to make some observations in order to classify these creatures.

(Show the students Sybil's creatures on the overhead projector and discuss characteristics that Sybil might observe in them.)

Sybil only had four cages in which to put the creatures. She wanted to develop a way of organizing the creatures so that not only would they fit in her four cages but so all the creatures in each cage would be alike in some way. Sybil, like all scientists, is very patient. She knows that it may take many tries before she is able to find a way or rule that works.

To get started Sybil makes an educated guess, which scientists call a **hypothesis**. Sybil wrote the hypothesis in her science journal. She tried to put the creatures in the cages according to how many feet they had.

(Label the cages 6 feet, 4 feet, 2 feet, and no feet. As you begin to put creatures into the cages, students will realize that some of the creatures have 1 or 3 feet. Since there is no place for these creatures, this hypothesis does not work.)

Sybil discovered that her hypothesis was not going to work. She did not have enough cages for all the different number of feet. What a unique group of creatures she had found!

(At this point have the students offer other suggestions about how to group the creatures back into the cages. There is no one right answer for classifying the laboratory creatures. Once the class has discovered a way of putting the creatures in the

cages finish reading the story. If no possible way is found, use the alternate ending.)

After successfully classifying all of the newly found creatures, Sybil sat down to record in her science journal her observations and her final rules for classifying the creatures. Since Sybil had tried many hypotheses before she found one that worked, she was very tired but very happy when she finally finished with her journal.

ALTERNATE ENDING

Sybil was not discouraged that she had not found a way that would work to sort and classify these creatures. She knew she could sleep on it that night and would certainly have a new idea for tomorrow.

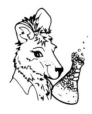

Sybil's Magnifying Glass

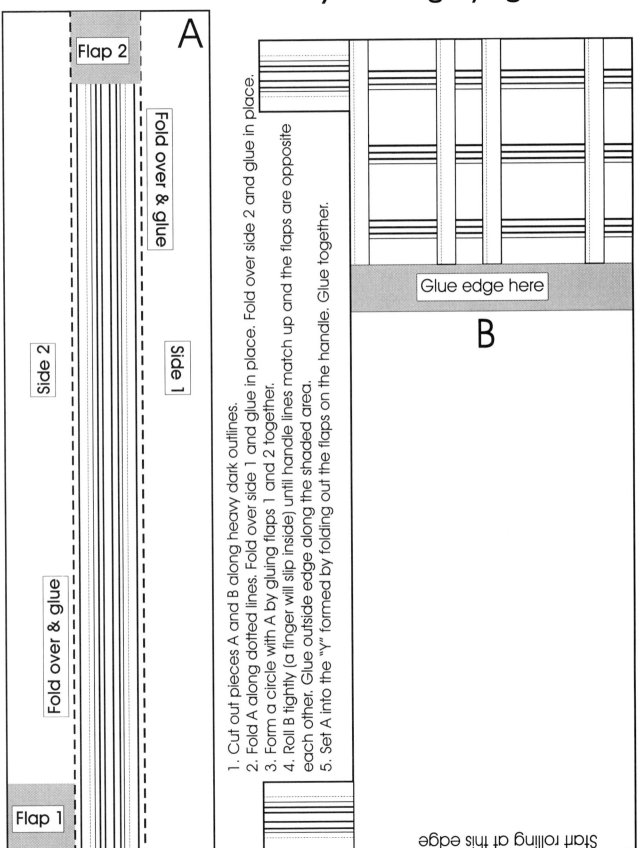

A

Flap 2

Fold over & glue

Side 2

Side 1

Fold over & glue

Flap 1

1. Cut out pieces A and B along heavy dark outlines.
2. Fold A along dotted lines. Fold over side 1 and glue in place. Fold over side 2 and glue in place.
3. Form a circle with A by gluing flaps 1 and 2 together.
4. Roll B tightly (a finger will slip inside) until handle lines match up and the flaps are opposite each other. Glue outside edge along the shaded area.
5. Set A into the "Y" formed by folding out the flaps on the handle. Glue together.

Glue edge here

B

Start rolling at this edge

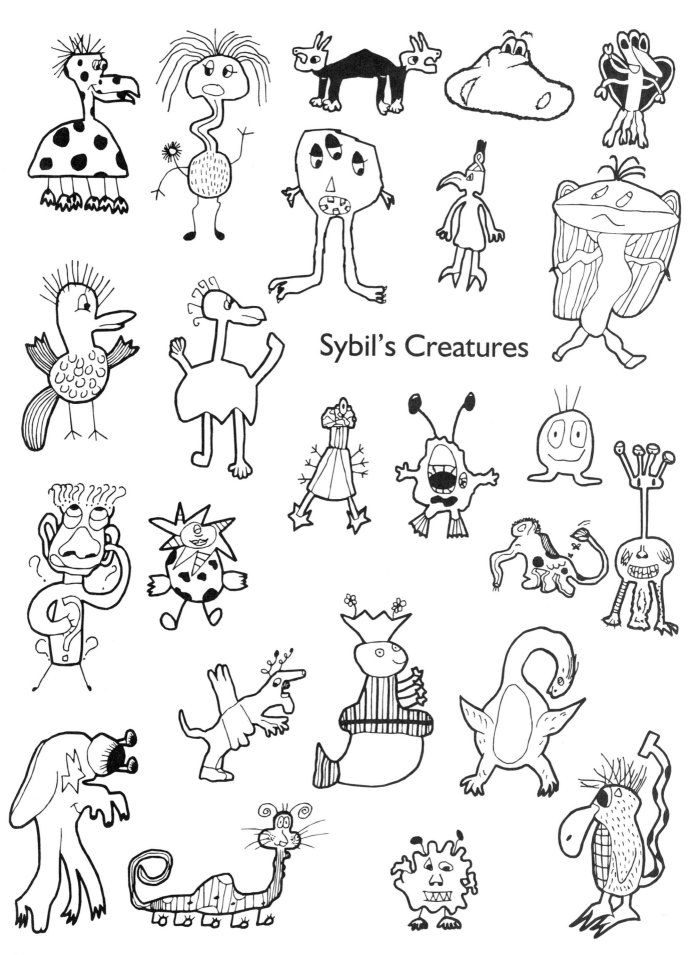

Sybil's Creatures

Sybil's Laboratory

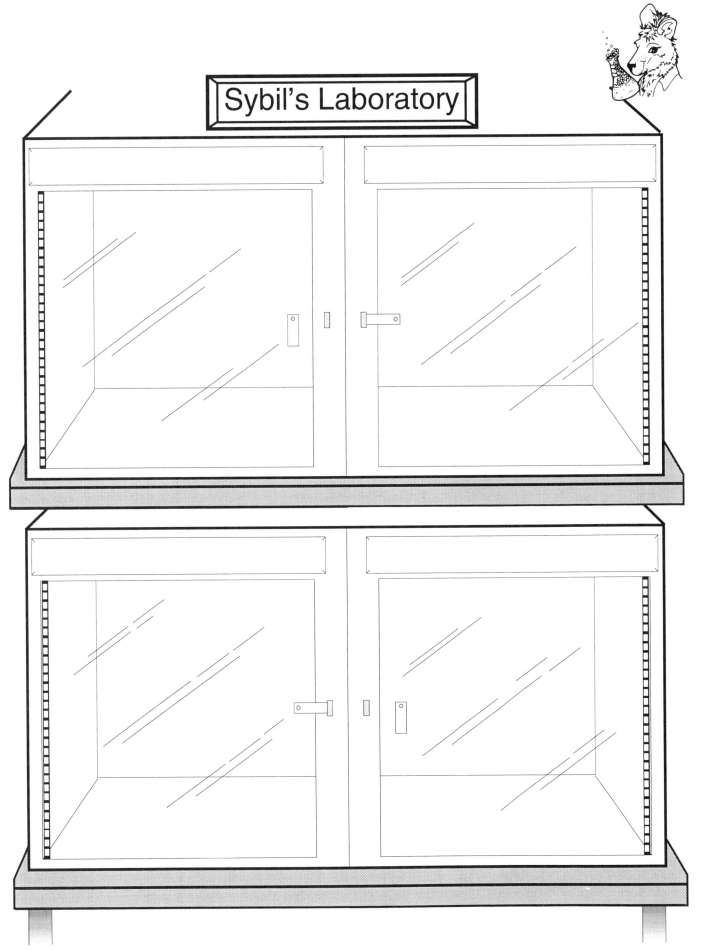

Loose Laboratory Limpets

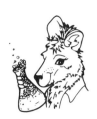

Help put these limpets back in their cages in Sybil's laboratory. Cut them out, group them, and glue them into their cages. Thanks!

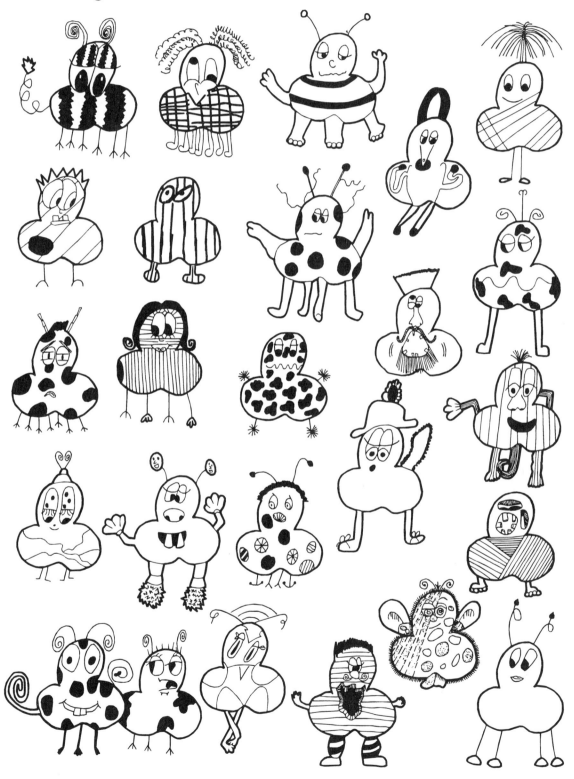

Name _____

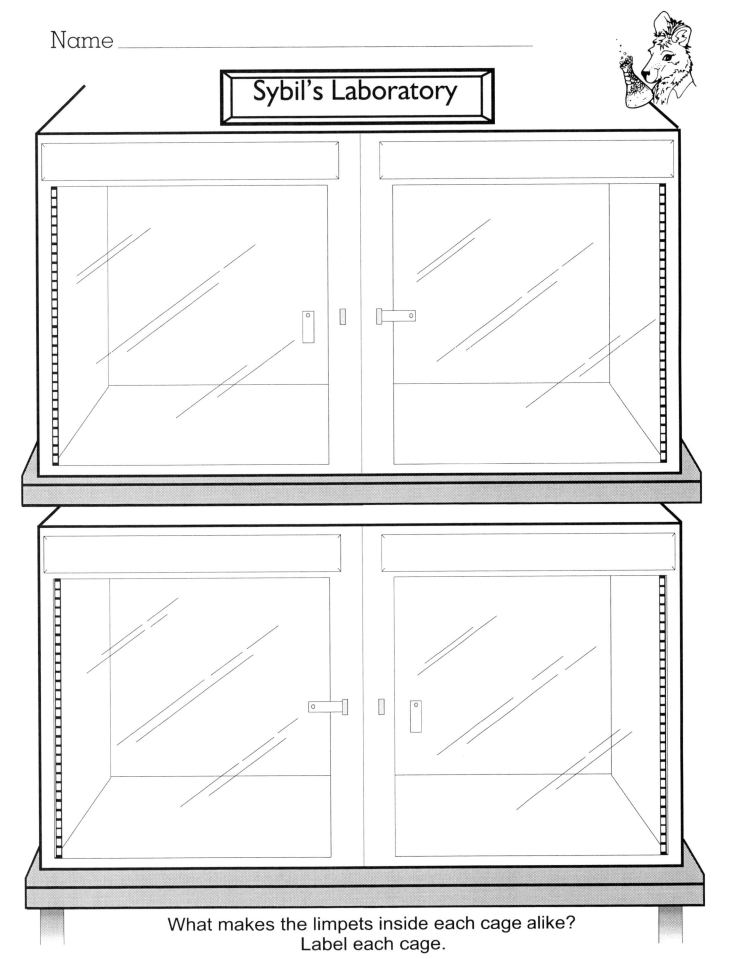

Sybil's Laboratory

What makes the limpets inside each cage alike?
Label each cage.

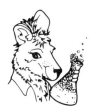

SCIENTIST THINKING
WHOLE CLASS
LESSON 2

PURPOSE

In this lesson, students will be introduced to another type of **analytical thinking: compare and contrast.** The lesson is designed as a class discussion.

TEACHER MATERIALS

— overhead transparencies of *Sybil's Scientific Pairs* and *More Scientific Pairs*
— a duplicated class set of *Thinking about Alike and Different*
— the Behavioral Checklist - *Scientist Thinking*

STUDENT MATERIALS

— crayons or markers
— pencils

LESSON PLAN

1. Review with students the concepts introduced in Lesson 1. A scientist loves to *classify and organize* information.

2. This lesson involves looking at two things and trying to determine how they are alike and how they are different. Put the overhead transparency *Sybil's Scientific Pairs* on the overhead projector. Ask students to suggest ways a button and a zipper are alike. As students provide answers, record them on the overhead transparencies. Follow this same procedure for comparing and contrasting a backpack and a lunch box. Additional comparison activities are provided and titled *More Scientific Pairs.*

CHALLENGE PAGE

Thinking about Alike and Different

3. *Thinking about Alike and Different* worksheets are provided as Challenge Pages. The teacher may want to give the *Thinking About Alike and Different* a page at a time to those students who are most interested.

DIAGNOSTIC NOTES

Look for students who are able to analytically compare and contrast. Also look for students who are able to do so in a creative or unusual way.

A checklist for the whole class lesson is provided. The following is a short summary of what to look for in student behaviors.

IDENTIFIES ATTRIBUTES - Look for students who understand the concept of attributes. They understand that similarly shaped shadows is a common attribute.

CREATES CLASSIFICATION SYSTEMS - Look for students who are able to create a classification system. This lesson does not offer as many opportunities to observe this characteristic as Whole Class Lesson 1.

DEMONSTRATES UNIQUE STRATEGIES - Look for students who find unique or unusual ways in which two things are alike or different.

DEFERS JUDGMENT - Look for students who are able to change course and try new ideas. These students may think of ideas for previous pairs after the class has gone ahead.

CURIOSITY AND KNOWLEDGE ABOUT SCIENCE - Look for students who know or want to know specific facts about science. Some students will bring to class a vast knowledge about science topics. This in itself does not indicate a potentially talented student, but combined with some of the other characteristics, will give the teacher a more complete picture of the student's potential.

LONG ATTENTION SPAN - Look for students who are willing to stick with the task even when the task is very difficult.

Thinking about Alike and Different
Look for students who are willing and able to complete many of the Challenge Pages. Creativity and the analytical aspect of comparing and contrasting should be noted.

NOTES

Sybil's Scientific Pairs

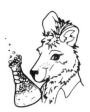

Sybil enjoys thinking scientifically about the world around her. Often she will think about how two things are alike and different. Help Sybil decide how these pairs are alike and different.

How is a button like a zipper?

_____

_____

How are they different?

_____

_____

How is a backpack like a lunch box?

_____

How are they different?

_____

_____

More Scientific Pairs

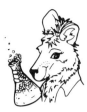

How is a rain forest like a circus?

_____

_____

_____

How are they different?

_____

_____

_____

How is a stamp like a good book?

_____

_____

_____

How are they different?

_____

_____

_____

More Scientific Pairs

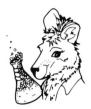

How is a fairy tale like a song?

_____

_____

How are they different?

_____

_____

How is the wind like a movie?

_____

_____

How are they different?

_____

_____

More Scientific Pairs

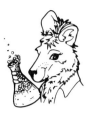

How is a seashell like a tree?

_____

_____

_____

How are they different?

_____

_____

_____

How is a door like friendship?

_____

_____

_____

How are they different?

_____

_____

_____

Name _____

Thinking about Alike and Different

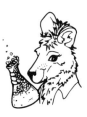

Alike		**Different**

Name _____

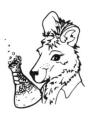

Thinking about Alike and Different

Alike   **Different**

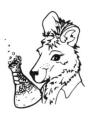

Name _____

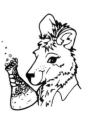

Thinking about Alike and Different

Alike		**Different**

Name _____

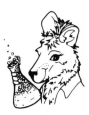

Thinking about Alike and Different

Alike		Different

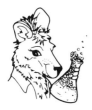

SCIENTIST THINKING
SMALL GROUP
LESSON 1

PURPOSE

The purpose of this lesson is to allow capable students further experiences in **analytical thinking**. They will practice the observation and classification skills that a scientist uses.

TEACHER MATERIALS

— a *Curiosity Caboodle* for each student or pair of students. The Lesson Plan provides further information about the *Curiosity Caboodle*.
— a duplicated classroom set of *Curiosity Caboodles: What's So Unusual?*
— a duplicated classroom set of *Curiosity Caboodles: Sort It*

STUDENT MATERIALS

— crayons
— pencils
— scissors
— magnifying glass

LESSON PLAN

1. For the small group activity, each student or pair of students will need a *Curiosity Caboodle.* The *Curiosity Caboodle* is just a collection of stuff in a self-sealing plastic bag. The teacher may choose to put the bags together using sorting items such as buttons, shells, marbles, or rocks. The teacher may also choose to have students put together a bag from home. Items could represent a theme such as "backyard stuff" or could be just a collection of "stuff." If students are to collect the items for the *Curiosity Caboodle,* the following is a sample letter that could be sent to parents:

Dear Parents,

We have an exciting opportunity to stimulate scientific thinking, but we need your help. The enclosed bag is for a *Curiosity Caboodle.* Please find at least 20 interesting items that will fit in the bag.

(At this point, discuss any theme items that are to be collected.)

2. Give each student or pair of students a *Curiosity Caboodle.* Ask students to look carefully at the objects in their bags. To observe objects more closely, students should use a magnifying glass.

3. Give each student a copy of *Curiosity Caboodles: What's So Unusual?* Students are to choose the two most unusual items from their bags. On the worksheet they are to describe each item in words and to draw pictures of the items.

4. For the second activity, students are to find a way to classify the items into groups so that the items in each group are alike in some way. After finding a way to sort the items, students should write or tell what is special about each group. The worksheet *Curiosity Caboodles: Sort It* is provided for students to record their groups and descriptions. An example of what a student might do is group all of the items made of wood. The special rule would be "made of wood."

5. The activity can be extended by re-sorting the same objects with a different set of rules or by trading bags.

DIAGNOSTIC NOTES

Look for students who are able to change when they realize their grouping will not work. Some students will stay with a bad choice, whereas others easily adjust to have successful groups. Look for students who are able to rearrange the objects numerous ways. Also note students who use creative or unusual ways of sorting.

NOTES

Name _____

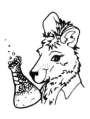

Curiosity Caboodles:
What's So Unusual?

- -

Item #1

_____

_____

_____

_____

_____

_____

- -

Item #2

_____

_____

_____

_____

_____

Name _____

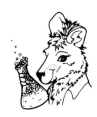

Curiosity Caboodles:
Sort It!

The things in this group _____

_____

_____

_____

_____

_____

_____

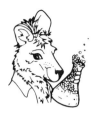

SCIENTIST THINKING
SMALL GROUP
LESSON 2

PURPOSE

The purpose of this lesson is to provide students with the opportunity to examine various aspects of objects, pair them, and then find another pair that has the same relationship. This activity requires both creative and analytical thinking as students arrange the cards according to **analogies.**

TEACHER MATERIALS

— a set of *Sybil's Picture Analogy Deck* or the group or for each pair of students
— large construction paper for students to glue the cards on

STUDENT MATERIALS

— scissors
— glue

LESSON PLAN

1. Introduce students to the concept of *analogies* by providing some simple examples. The following are some possibilities:

> hand is to glove as foot is to shoe
> green is to grass as brown is to dirt

Ask students to brainstorm some of their own analogies to be sure they understand.

2. This activity can be done as a group activity, in pairs, or individually. If the entire group works together, this allows interesting discussion. The teacher may hear ideas and observe behaviors which provide more insight than if students work individually. Having students work in pairs provides opportunities for discussion and more participation.

3. The *Sybil's Picture Analogy Deck* allows for a variety of matchings. Some matchings are more obvious than others. Similar, opposite, action of the objects, characteristics, whole to part, object to group or mathematical relationships are some of the matchings possible in the cards. Show students the deck of cards but do not tell them the possible relationships. Remind students that the order is important. For example, if the analogy is

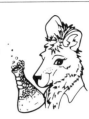

"*cat* is to kitten as *dog* is to puppy"

it is important for the adult animals to be first on both sides.

4. Students can glue their analogies to the construction paper. Encourage students to wait until the very end before gluing on their cards. As students begin to match analogy cards, they may realize that if they change some of their earlier matches, they are able to use more of the cards.

5. Depending on the student's viewpoint, cards can be combined in a variety of ways. Some combinations may not be obvious, requiring an explanation from the student. Accept any analogy that offers a reasonable relationship. If no reasonable combination of cards can be found to complete the second part of the analogy, then the first part of the relationship and possibly other already completed analogies must be regrouped to make a larger number of correct analogies.

DIAGNOSTIC NOTES

If this activity is being used as a diagnostic tool, listening to the reasoning is just as important as keeping track of the number of reasonable combinations expressed in the correct order. Look for students who are able to put together analogies. Also look for students who are able to use the correct **A:B::C:D** order. Note students who are willing to change previous analogies in order to find a better fit. This activity provides teachers with an opportunity to note creative and unusual analogies.

NOTES

Sybil's Picture Analogy Card Deck

green

STOP

red

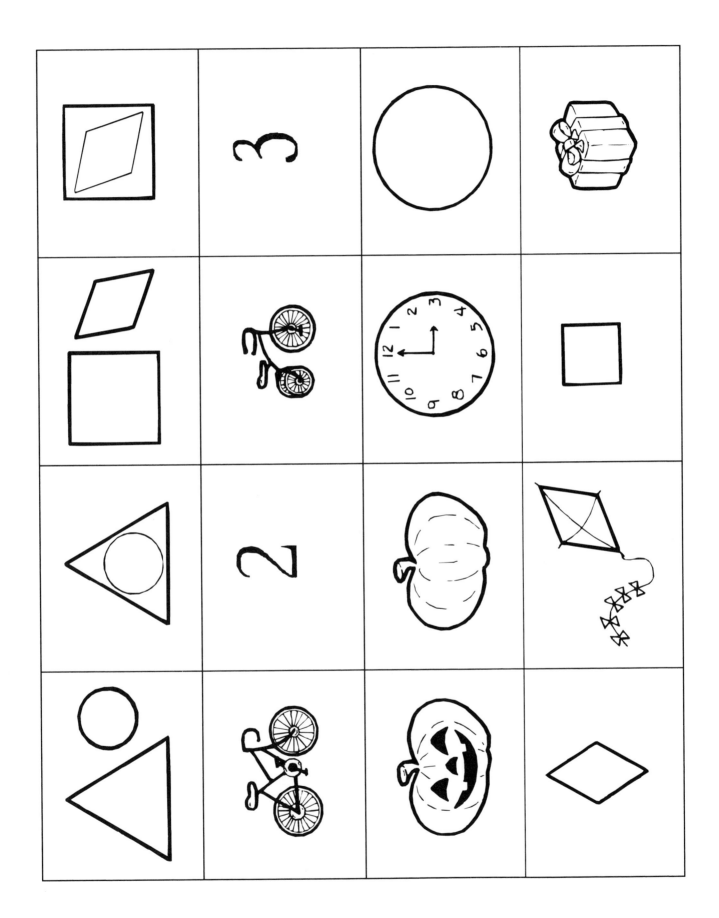

pan		4	
nap			10
321		8	
123			5

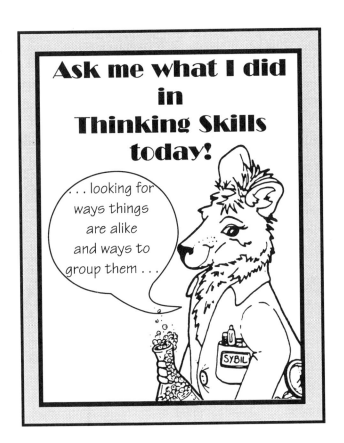

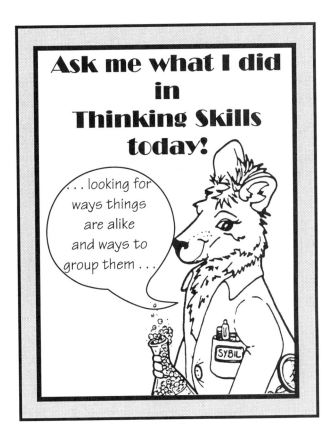

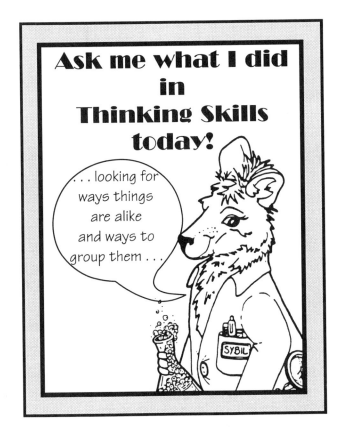

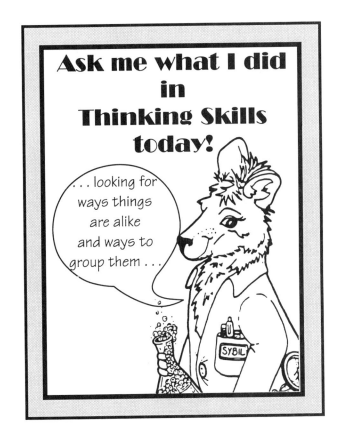

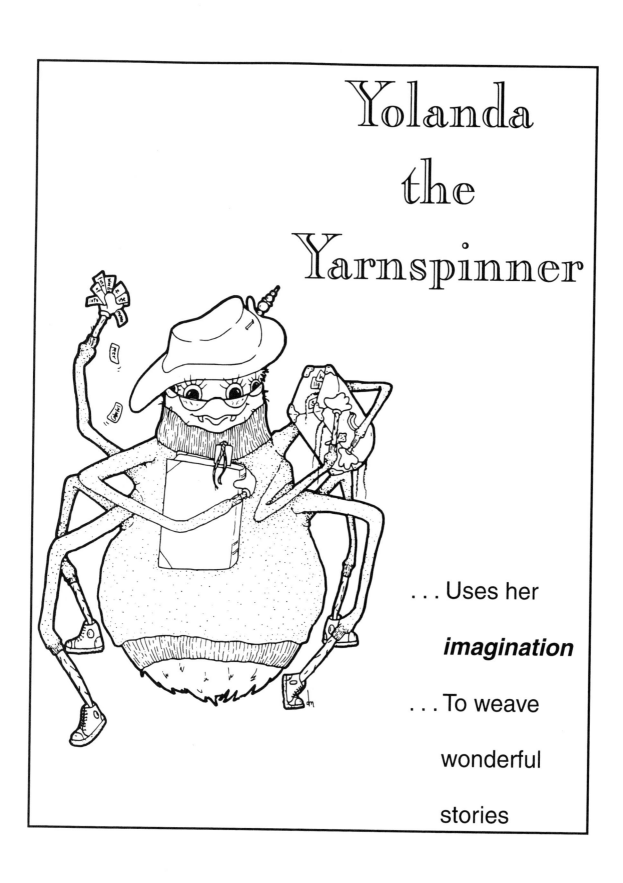

Yolanda the Yarnspinner

. . . Uses her

imagination

. . . To weave

wonderful

stories

Yolanda the Yarnspinner

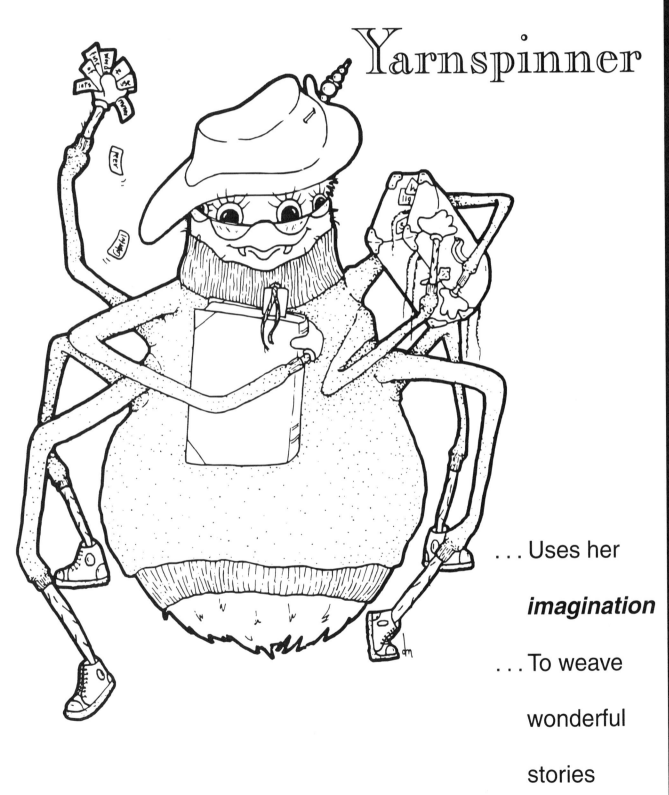

Divergent / Creative Thinking

. . . Uses her

imagination

. . . To weave

wonderful

stories

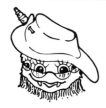

YARNSPINNER THINKING
WHOLE CLASS
LESSON 1

PURPOSE

The purpose of this lesson is to review and reinforce the concepts for **divergent thinking**. As students learn about the art of storytelling, they will meet *Yolanda the Yarnspinner* character who makes colorful word pictures with her divergent thoughts. Students will learn that in divergent thinking:

— There are many possibilities.
— Ideas may begin from a common "stem" but branch in different directions from there.
— A creative imagination helps us see many possibilities in ordinary events, situations, and objects.

TEACHER MATERIALS

— one copy of the *Yolanda the Yarnspinner* story to read aloud to students
— an overhead transparency of the picture of *Yolanda the Yarnspinner* and/or a class set of duplicated pictures for students to color
— black yarn
— a duplicated set of *Yolanda's Bookmarks* for students
— a set of colored overhead transparency markers
— an overhead transparency of *Skeletal Sentences*
— a blank transparency
— a duplicated class set of *Stupendous Statements*
— Behavioral Checklist - *Storyteller Thinking*

STUDENT MATERIALS

— crayons or markers
— pencils
— glue
— scissors

LESSON PLAN

1. Introduce students to the lesson by asking if they have ever told a story. If so, they are *storytellers*. Ask students what characteristics make a good storyteller. Hopefully students will respond with *imagination, creativity,* and *interesting ideas*. Some story-tellers write their stories and others tell their stories. Ask students what some of their favorite stories are.

2. Explain to students that today they are going to meet *Yolanda the Yarnspinner* who uses her creative imagination to tell colorful stories. Show them the picture of Yolanda (page 114) on the overhead projector. You may wish to have them color the pictures of Yolanda (page 115) at this time or following the reading of Yolanda's story.

3. Read *Yolanda the Yarnspinner* story.

4. Review with the students these points from the story:

— A good storyteller uses words in creative ways to make entertaining pictures in our minds.
— There are many possibilities in storytelling, but the ideas need to match the story "stem."
— Good storytellers love to play with words, and they enjoy searching for just the right word to make their word pictures perfect.

5. Give students one of Yolanda's bookmarks and pieces of yarn to glue onto the bookmark. The bookmark is the memory trigger for this unit to help students remember to think like a storyteller during their activities.

6. To practice making sentences more colorful, a list of *Skeletal Sentences* (subject - verb only) have been provided. These can be copied onto overhead transparencies and the individual words cut out to use on the overhead projector. Ask the students to expand the sentences and make them colorful by answering the questions you ask about the sentences. Write their responses on an overhead transparency in a variety of colored inks to illustrate the concept that you are using colorful words to make the sentences grow.

For Example: Place the sentence *"The boy ran."* on the overhead. Each word should be cut out on a short strip of transparency film. This will make it easier to move the words around as students add colorful words. Ask the students questions such as these:
- Is this a complete sentence? *(Yes, it is, because it has the requisite parts: a subject and a verb. But we can make this sentence more colorful by thinking like Yolanda.)*
- What kind of boy was he? *(Accept any reasonable response, and use a colored marker to insert the response between "The" and "boy.")*
- Where did he run? *(Again, accept any reasonable response, and use another colored marker to insert the response in the appropriate spot.)*
- How was he running? *(Accept reasonable adverbs and place in the appropriate place in the sentence with a different colored marker.)*
- Why was he running there? *(This phrase will most likely end the sentence, but you may continue questioning in this manner until you have a sentence you think is colorful, sensible, and complete.)*

Have the students notice all the colors they were able to add to this sentence. You may use all the sentences provided, use just a few, or create your own.

CHALLENGE PAGES

Stupendous Statements

7. Distribute the Challenge Pages. The Challenge Pages will give teachers an opportunity to observe an aspect of the divergent thinking process. When doing the Challenge Pages, students may choose to use the words more than once. The most important aspect of the Challenge Pages is the type of sentence students write.

DIAGNOSTIC NOTES

The characteristics to be looked for in this lesson are very similar to the Inventor Thinking, which is also divergent thinking:

MANY IDEAS - Look for students who are able to supply many ideas.

COLORFUL WORDS - Look for students who are able to use colorful words and original responses to create a visual image.

PHRASES - Look for students who use phrases rather than single words. This shows the ability to elaborate with words.

ORIGINAL RESPONSES - Look for students who are able to give you ideas that are original or unusual.

SENSE OF HUMOR - This unit offers opportunity for students to incorporate humor. Look for those students with a subtle or advanced sense of humor.

ADVANCED VOCABULARY - Look for students who correctly use a large vocabulary. Also look for students who can express themselves in a mature, articulate manner.

Stupendous Statements
Look for students who can put the words together to form many responses. Note those students who can make sentences which display an unusual or advanced sense of humor. Also look for students who can use many of the words in one sentence. It is not very creative for a student to write *"I have a fast cat."* and then follow it by *"I have a fast, fast cat."* and so on. Look for students who are able to put together a variety of different sentences.

P E T S

List names of students as each behavior appears. Add checkmarks after name if behavior is repeated. Use a different color of ink or pencil for each whole group lesson.	**Behavioral Checklist** ---------- **Yarnspinner Thinking** (Creative Thinking/Divergent)	Teacher _____ Grade: 1 ___ 2 ___ 3 ___ Dates of whole 1. _____ group instruction: 2. _____

OFFERS MANY IDEAS (fluency)	*USES COLORFUL WORDS* (flexibility) TO CREATE VISUAL IMAGES
USES PHRASES RATHER THAN SINGLE WORDS (elaboration) TO EXPRESS IDEAS	*OFFERS ORIGINAL RESPONSES* (originality) TO CREATE VISUAL IMAGES
DISPLAYS AN UNUSUAL/MATURE *SENSE OF HUMOR*	*USES ADVANCED VOCABULARY;* CAN EXPRESS SELF IN A MATURE, ARTICULATE MANNER
PETS classwork indicates an outstanding ability to use this thinking skill.	The following student/s did not participate during the thinking skills lessons, but I see these behaviors during **regular class time**.

YOLANDA THE YARNSPINNER

On a bright, sunny day in Crystal Pond Woods, Yolanda the Yarnspinner was in her tree doing her second favorite thing, spinning a beautiful web. As she was spinning away, that mischievous raccoon, Rascal Raccoon, came running up.

"Yolanda, Yolanda!" he yelled. "Please, help me. I need your help."

Yolanda stopped spinning her web and looked down at Rascal Raccoon. She could not imagine why he would need her help, but she was polite enough not to say so.

"Of course I will help you," said Yolanda, "if I can."

"The most exciting thing has happened to me, and I want to share it at the community campfire tonight," said Rascal Raccoon. "I am afraid that once I start telling the story, I will get nervous, and it will not sound nearly as exciting. Please, Yolanda, please help me with my story. Everyone in Crystal Pond Woods knows that you are the best at spinning yarns."

Rascal Raccoon was correct. Yolanda is known far and wide as one of the best yarnspinners. It is her favorite thing to do. **Spinning yarns** is another way of saying she is a storyteller. The creatures of Crystal Pond Woods love to listen to Yolanda spin her stories. One reason Yolanda is very good at telling stories is that she has a very creative imagination. She can turn everyday activities or objects into an entertaining web of magic. Sometimes her stories are make-believe, and sometimes they are real, but they are always entertaining.

Another reason Yolanda is so good at spinning yarns is that she knows a lot of words. She always searches for just the right word to put magic into her story. In her trunk of yarns, Yolanda has all kinds of words. She has words that rhyme, words that imitate sounds, and words that begin with the same sound. She uses words to paint pictures that you can see clearly in your mind. Yolanda is an artist with words.

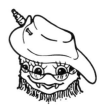

Rascal Raccoon had certainly picked the right friend for help!

Yolanda reached into her trunk and drew out some yarn. She finds it very helpful to her creative process if she winds yarn while she thinks of her story. Sometimes Yolanda would spin her yarn to make a bookmark. Even though Yolanda is a storyteller, she loves to read other people's stories and can always use a good bookmark. After choosing the yarn, Yolanda began to make her bookmark. She offered yarn to Rascal Raccoon so he could make a bookmark. Now Yolanda was ready to help Rascal Raccoon.

"First," she said, "tell me about the exciting thing that happened to you."

"Well," started Rascal Raccoon, "early this morning I went through Dudley the Detective's yard, saw his open window, and climbed in through the window. There I saw Rosalyn Robin take Dudley's badge! Then I climbed out the window, ran through the backyard, and climbed over the fence."

"You are right, Rascal Raccoon," Yolanda replied. "You saw something very exciting, but you are not using exciting words to describe what happened to you. I will help you spin a more colorful story. First, what kind of morning was it?"

"It was a bright, sunny morning," answered Rascal Raccoon.

"Bright and sunny are colorful words. Be sure that you include those words when you tell your story," said Yolanda. "What did Dudley's yard look like?"

"His yard was very shiny because of the dew on the ground," replied Rascal Raccoon.

Yolanda knew the perfect word for Rascal Raccoon to use to describe the yard. "The yard **sparkled** in the sunlight," she suggested.

Rascal Raccoon was very impressed. Yolanda was very good with words.

"What made you look at Dudley's window?" continued Yolanda.

"Well," said Rascal Raccoon, "the curtains were flying out of the window blowing in the wind."

"Hmmm," murmured Yolanda as she wound yarn around her pencil. "The curtains were **billowing** in the wind."

"Wow, Yolanda," cried Rascal Raccoon. "It was a bright, sunny morning. The yard **sparkled** in the sunlight. Dudley the Detective's curtains were **billowing** in the wind. Rosalyn Robin's wings **swished** as she flew in the window. I thought of "swish" because that is how the wings sounded as she flew."

"You are doing great!" exclaimed Yolanda. "You are very creative. What happened after Rosalyn Robin flew in the window?"

"I climbed in the window and saw her take Dudley the Detective's badge. Then she flew to her nest in the apple tree," continued Rascal Raccoon.

"I know we can think of a few colorful words to use," said Yolanda as she spun her yarn. "Why don't you use **peered** instead of looked. What did Dudley's badge look like?"

"Well, it was **shiny** and **gold**. I think I'm beginning to get the idea, Yolanda. When I tell my story, I should try to use words that will paint a picture of what I saw," said Rascal Raccoon.

"You are going to be a great storyteller at the community campfire tonight. I can't wait to hear your entire story," replied Yolanda.

"Yolanda, I need to go practice my story. Is it okay if I keep the yarn bookmark to remind me of all the different kinds of words I can use in my story?" asked Rascal Raccoon.

"Yes," said Yolanda, "Tonight I will be cheering you on as you tell your exciting story. Good Luck!" Yolanda waved good-bye to Rascal Raccoon with four of her eight legs.

Yolanda's Bookmarks

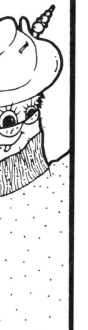

Cut out the bookmarks. Decorate Yolanda's sweater with pieces of yarn glued in place. Be sure to allow 8 pieces to dangle from the bottom — Yolanda's legs, of course!

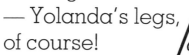

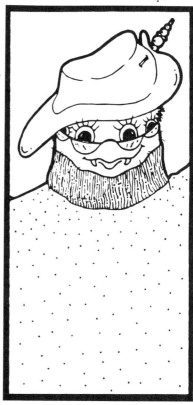

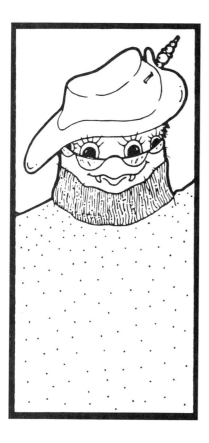

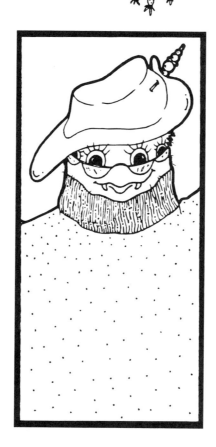

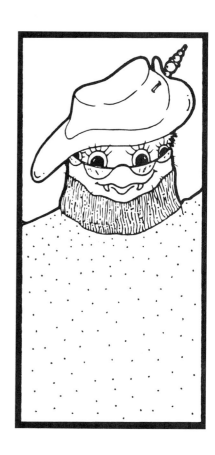

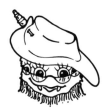

"Skeletal Sentences"

The boy ran

My mother reads

The dog barked

Our house sits

The baby is crying

Name _____

Stupendous Statements

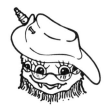

Use only the words below to write as many sentences as you can. Your sentences can be silly or serious.

I	cat	paper	on	with
door	play	have	and	has
a	to	fast	will	can

_____

_____

_____

_____

_____

_____

_____

_____

Name _____

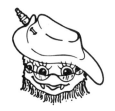

Stupendous Statements

Use only the words below to write as many sentences as you can. Be creative — you may be silly or serious.

I	a	was	hamburger
ate	tiger	car	in	eat
have	to	and	fast	going

_____

_____

_____

_____

_____

_____

_____

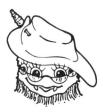

YARNSPINNER THINKING
WHOLE CLASS
LESSON 2

PURPOSE

The purpose of this lesson is to review and reinforce the concepts of creative thinking in the **storytelling** process by incorporating a **pattern** into the students' stories. Since in the creative process, thoughts may begin from a common stem but branch divergently from there, students will be asked to create a story using a pattern demonstrated during the lesson. Students will review these concepts:

— In creative thinking there are many possibilities.
— Ideas branch divergently from a common stem.
— A creative imagination is a useful tool for a storyteller.
— Storytelling incorporates colorful words and phrasing.

TEACHER MATERIALS

— one copy of either book **Fortunately** by Remy Charlip or **That's Good** by Margery Cuyler
— an overhead transparency of *Good News! Bad News!*
— a duplicated class set of blank *What Good News! What Bad News!*
— optional duplicated sets of *Making News* for capable writers
— Behavioral checklist - *Yarnspinner Thinking*

STUDENT MATERIALS

— crayons
— pencils

LESSON PLAN

1. Review with students the concepts for divergent thinking related to *storytelling*. Students learned in the previous lesson that there are many possibilities for stories and although ideas may begin from a common stem they can branch in different directions. A creative imagination sees many possibilities in ordinary events, situations, and objects.

2. Read aloud to the students the book **Fortunately** by Remy Charlip or **That's Good! That's Bad!** by Margery Cuyler. Ask students to describe any pattern they see in the story, either in the words or in the illustrations. Ask them also to identify any words or phrases which they found particularly colorful.

3. Following the reading of the story and its discussion, read the sample *Good News! Bad News!* transparency with the students. Ask them to use their creative thinking to write their own original stories which follow the *Good News/Bad News* pattern on the blank *What Good News! What Bad News!* page. Remind them to make good use of colorful words and phrases wherever possible. Capable students might do the more difficult Challenge Pages *Making News* instead or as an additional follow up. The *Making News* pages are a set in which students must plan ahead to incorporate an unusual prompt into the middle of a *Good News/Bad News* story. Developing a smooth flow throughout presents the students with an exceptional challenge.

DIAGNOSTIC NOTES

The characteristics to be looked for in this lesson are very similar to the Inventor Thinking, which is also divergent thinking.

MANY IDEAS - Look for students who are able to supply many ideas.

COLORFUL WORDS - Look for students who are able to use colorful words and original responses to create a visual image.

PHRASES - Look for students who use phrases rather than single words. This shows the ability to elaborate with words.

ORIGINAL RESPONSES - Look for students who are able to give you ideas that are original or unusual.

SENSE OF HUMOR - This unit offers opportunity for students to incorporate humor. Look for those students with a subtle or advanced sense of humor.

ADVANCED VOCABULARY - Look for students who correctly utilize a large vocabulary. Also look for students who can express themselves in a mature, articulate manner.

NOTES

Good News! Bad News!

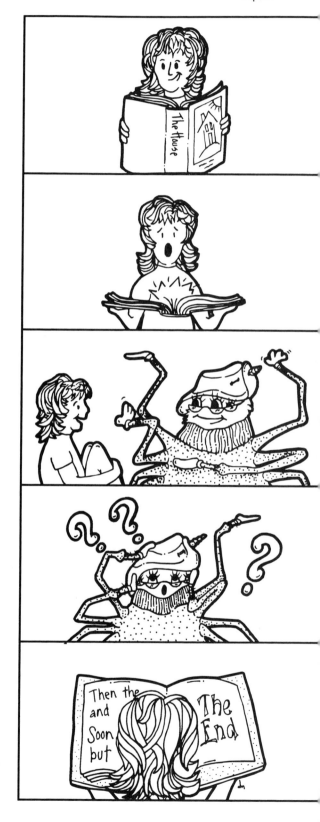

1. Good news!

   Mary has a new storybook.

2. Bad news!

   Some pages are missing!

3. Good news!

   Yolanda knows this story.

4. Bad news!

   Yolanda forgot the ending!

5. Good news!

   Mary can read the
   ending in the book. Those
   pages are there!

Name _____

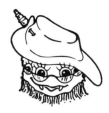

What Good News!
What Bad News!

1. Good news!

2. Bad news!

3. Good news!

4. Bad news!

5. Good news!

Name _____

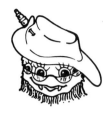

Making News

Write the missing lines and draw pictures for this news story.

WHAT GOOD NEWS!

My cousin is coming over to play.

WHAT BAD NEWS!

_____

Name _____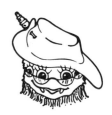

WHAT GOOD NEWS!

There is ice cream in the freezer.

WHAT BAD NEWS!

_____

Name _____

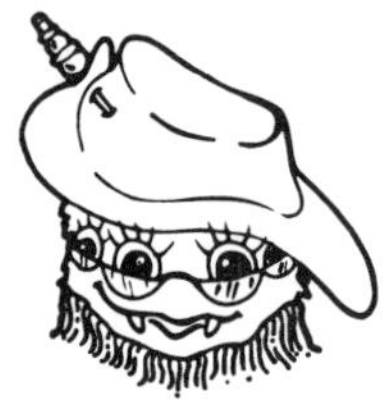

WHAT GOOD NEWS!

_____

AND, WHAT GOOD NEWS!

_____

YARNSPINNER THINKING
SMALL GROUP
LESSON 1

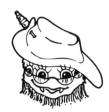

PURPOSE

The purpose of this lesson is to give students the opportunity to display their creative thinking with **word play**. Based on the work of Dr. E. Paul Torrance, the creative thinker is one who displays fluency, flexibility, originality, and elaboration. In addition, many researchers feel that one identifier of gifted students is an advanced sense of humor. This lesson provides the students with an outlet for all these traits.

TEACHER MATERIALS

— a chalkboard, overhead, or chart paper for brainstorming
— a large piece of chart paper for recording students' final riddles
   OR
— a duplicated class set of *Radical Riddles*

STUDENT MATERIALS

— pencils (if using worksheet)

LESSON PLAN

1. Students are going to write *riddles* about animals. Have them think of an animal, such as a pig. Next they list all the one-syllable words that go with this animal. Some examples might be *slop, ham, snout, boar, sow,* etc. Then they drop the first sound of this word. *Slop* would become *op, ham* becomes *am,* and so on.

The next step is to think of long words that begin with "op" or "am" or whatever. Then add the dropped sound to the beginning of the long word. A riddle then might be something like this: What do pigs do on their night out? Go to the "slopera!" Or: How do injured pigs get to the hospital? In a "hambulance!"

2. The brainstorming for this activity should be done as a group, with children helping one another for the best list of riddles. A variety of animals can be used.

3. Try to find a real audience for the riddles. Have students illustrate their riddles. These riddles often make an interesting bulletin board or can be part of the school newsletter or other published format.

DIAGNOSTIC NOTES

Look for students who understand and can perform the wordplay and enjoy doing so. Also note students who have lots of ideas. Having original ideas is also an important characteristic of potential talent. Also look for students who can change categories of thought. This is an area where an advanced sense of humor has an opportunity to shine.

NOTES

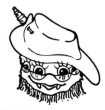

STUDENT RIDDLES

1. What do cows do in math class?

2. What do you call horses who wear masks and play baseball?

3. What do dogs go on when there is a flood?

4. What happens when a rabbit dials zero?

5. What do you call rabbits from outer space?

6. What do rabbit doctors perform?

7. Who makes the rules when rabbits play baseball?

8. What do you call a cow with a hard shell on its back?

9. What do pigs plug their TV's into?

10. What do cows wear in the battle?

11. What is a cat's favorite dessert?

12. Why do cows curl up and roll away?

13. Why do pigs go to the North Pole?

14. What do you call a doghouse designer?

15. How can you tell black bunnies from white bunnies?

16. When does cat's fur fall off?

Written by 1st graders at Husmann Elementary School, Crystal Lake, Illinois

16 Every claw-tumm!
15. Because they're hop-isites!
14. A bark-itecht!
13. To live in pig-loos!
12. Because they're pretending to be farm-adilloes!
11. Mice cream!
10. Suits of farm-our!
9. Squeal-ectric outlets!

8. A farm-adillo!
7. Major league jump-ires!
6. Hop-erations!
5. Cotton Taillens!
4. He gets the hop-erator!
3. Noah's Bark
2. Jump-ires!
1. Cud-dition facts

Name _____

Radical Riddles

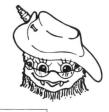

1. Think of an animal:

<table>
<tr><td></td></tr>
</table>

2. List 5 short words you can think of to go with this animal:

3. Drop the first sound of each word. List a long word that begins with what's left of the short word:

4. Add back the first sound of the short word to the long word:

_____

_____

_____

_____

_____

_____

_____

_____

_____

_____

_____

_____

_____

_____

_____

5. Now write some riddles about your animal:

6. Use the new long words as your answers:

YARNSPINNER THINKING
SMALL GROUP
LESSON 2

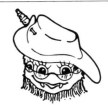

The purpose of this lesson is to review and reinforce the concepts of creative thinking in the *storytelling* process by incorporating a **pattern** into the students' stories. Since in the creative process, thoughts may begin from a common stem but branch divergently from there, students will be asked to create a poem using a pattern demonstrated during the lesson. Students will review these concepts:

— In creative thinking there are many possibilities.
— Ideas branch divergently from a common stem.
— A creative imagination is a useful tool for a storyteller.
— Storytelling incorporates colorful words and phrasing.

TEACHER MATERIALS

— chart paper and markers

STUDENT MATERIALS

— crayons (to illustrate the final product)

LESSON PLAN

1. Students will learn how to create *onomatopoeia* poems. Onomatopoetic words imitate the sound they describe. Examples include *boom, crunch,* and *drip.*

2. Students are going to use their sound words to write poems which describe a special place. The examples on the following page can be read to students.

OUR BAND

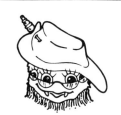

In the band you hear a drum
  BOOM! BOOM! BOOM!
Behind it is a little bell
  RING-DING-DING
The cymbals make a clanging sound
  CRASH! CRASH! CRASH!
The flutes can be heard all 'round
  TWITTER, TWITTER, TWEET

The music's beat makes my feet go
  TAP, TAP, TAP

And when it's done,
It's been such fun.
  CLAP! CLAP! CLAP!

Written by 1st graders at Husmann Elementary School, Crystal Lake, Illinois

NOISES AT THE ZOO

The noises at the zoo
They sound kind of like this.
"Roar," roared the great big lion.
"Eeek, eeek," giggled the furry monkeys.
"Hee, hee, haw, haw," laughed the hyenas.
"Growl," growled the grizzly bear.
"Hiss," hissed the king cobra.
"Screech," scratched the bob cat.
"Snap," snapped the jaws of the alligator.
*"S*queak," squeaked the gray mouse.
"Boom, boom, boom," went the elephant.
"Hush," said the zookeeper.

Written by first graders at Coventry Elementary School, Crystal Lake, Illinois

As the students were writing this poem, they tried to include colorful words as discussed in the Whole Class Lesson 1.

3. Have students brainstorm a list of words that sound like noises. The following are possible words to be used in the poems and can be referred to or added to the list brainstormed by students.

YOLANDA'S WORD BANK

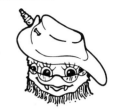

WORDS THAT SOUND LIKE NOISES - onomatopoeia

buzz	crash	sizzle	clink	squeak
slam	clank	rat-a-tat	bang	purr
hush	splash	chirp	tinkle	thump
clap	hiss	slosh	pop	clang
swoosh	jingle	roar	eeek	jangle

WORDS TO USE INSTEAD OF "SAID"

roar	sang	tweeter	screech	hoot
howl	giggle	rumble	cry	stomp
yip	purr	laugh	growl	scratch
grumble	squawk	squeal	chirp	bark
croak	titter	smack	chuckle	chortle
loud	quiet	soft	whisper	shout
blare	hiss	yell	stomp	thunder

4. Have students imagine a very noisy place (the school bandroom, a big city, a zoo, etc.). As a group, write a poem using onomatopoeia that describes this special place. As students dictate the poem in a group, record their dictation, perhaps on a large poster which could be illustrated and displayed or published. Students can follow any poetic form that brings the sounds of their "place" to life. The first line of the poem should help to establish the location of the poem, and subsequent lines should be used to help the reader "hear" the sounds of their noisy place.

DIAGNOSTIC NOTES

Look for students who grasp the concept of onomatopoeia. Also look for students who can list lots of onomatopoeia. Students with colorful phrasing, poetic bent, and advanced vocabulary, humor or ideas show potential.

NOTES

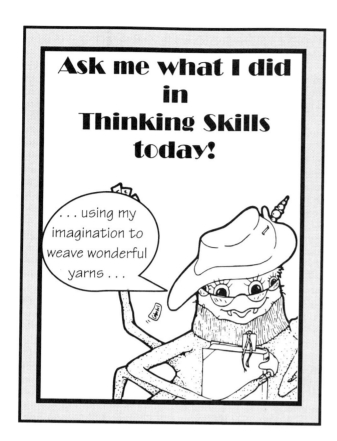

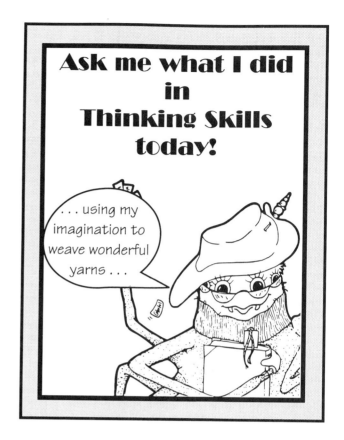

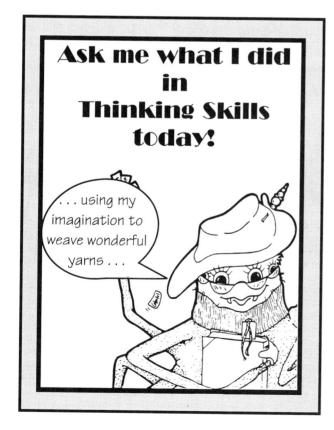

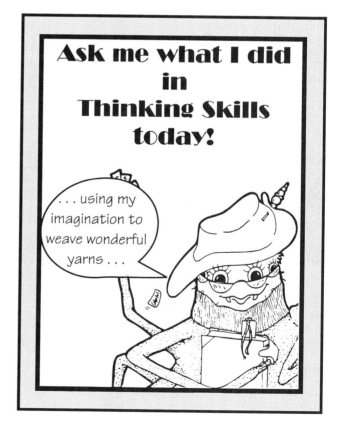

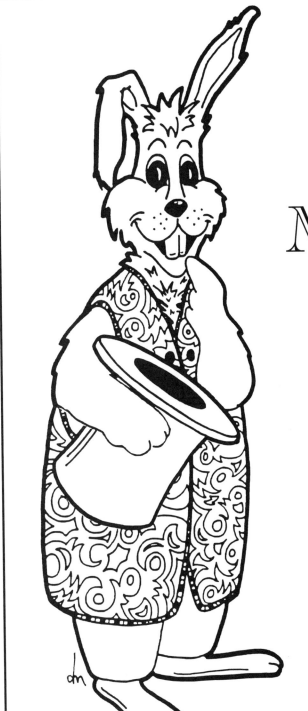

Max
the
Magician

. . . Looks for

patterns

. . . To find

one solution

that works

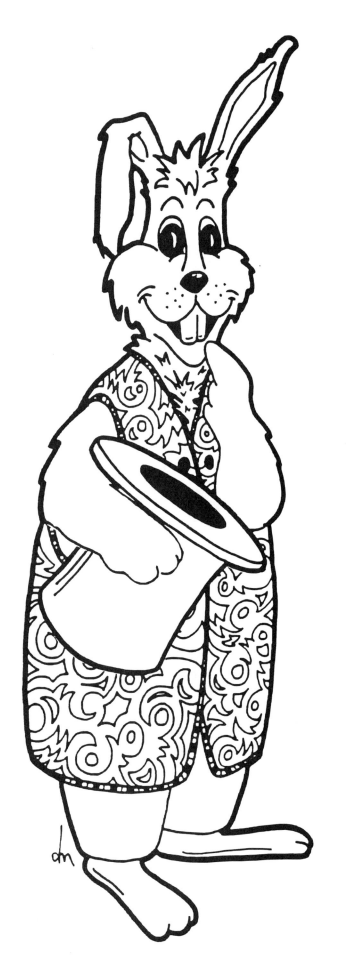

Max
the
Magician

. . . Looks for

patterns

. . . To find

one solution

that works

MAGICIAN THINKING
WHOLE CLASS
LESSON 1

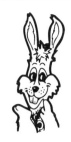

PURPOSE

The purpose of this lesson is to combine **analysis and synthesis** into an active thinking forum providing children with experiences to stimulate their **spatial intelligence**. In these activities, students will be introduced to *Max the Magician* who attempts to "fool our brains" through what our eyes perceive. This combines previously learned thinking skills in analyzing spatial relationships and reconstructing the parts into new wholes by making predictions. Students will be introduced to the following concepts:

— Thinking skills do not occur in isolation; spatial perception combines various thinking skills into the activities.
— Shapes can be manipulated mentally, without concrete devices.
— Visual patterns are predictable.
— The eyes and the brain must work together to "think" about given information.
— Tolerance for ambiguity and perseverance are essential components for flexible, high-level thinking skills.

TEACHER MATERIALS

— one copy of *Max the Magician* story
— an overhead transparency of the picture of *Max the Magician* and/or a class set of duplicated pictures for students to color
— an overhead transparency of *Max's Hatband*
— a set of pattern blocks for students and/or the overhead projector
— a duplicated class set of *Max's Magic Hat*
— green and red overhead transparency markers
— an overhead transparency of *Rabbit Reversal*
— an overhead transparency of *Designer Details*
— a duplicated class set of *Max's Hat Tricks*
— a duplicated class set of *Make Max Reappear*
— Behavioral Checklist - *Magician Thinking*

STUDENT MATERIALS

— pencils   — scissors
— crayons   — glue

LESSON PLAN

1. Introduce students to the concept of a *magician*. Magicians do not actually do magic. Instead they trick us by how we see or perceive things. Magicians are able to fool our eyes. Magicians appear to pull a quarter out of a person's ear. The brain knows that the quarter was not in the ear, but the eyes are fooled into believing the trick. When using magician thinking, the brain must work with the eyes to fill in the information that the eyes do not see.

2. Read the story *Max the Magician*. During the story, the teacher will need to put the transparency of *Max's Hatband* on the overhead. The triangles need to be colored green and the rectangles need to be colored red.

3. Have students make the pencil holder which is the thinking skill memory trigger for this unit.

4. Using a predictable three-dimensional object, such as a teddy bear, help the students understand how to visualize the sides of the object that are not facing them. Hold the teddy bear close to your chest so that the students cannot see the back of it. It is preferable that the teddy bear have several distinguishing marks about it (a hat, a scarf, posable arms and legs, etc). Ask the students to describe the bear to you. They will tell you about the bear's shape, color, hat, scarf and so on. Ask students to tell you what the back of the bear looks like. Do the stripes on the hat go all the way around to the back? Is the scarf tied around the bear's neck, or is it stitched on at the sides?

5. Discuss how the students can "see" with their minds what they cannot see with their eyes. Help them understand that while they cannot be 100% certain that the back of this brown bear is not purple or whether or not it has a tail (since it is not a real bear, but a stuffed toy), their brains help them fill in the logical details about what they can expect. If the bear has posable arms and legs, ask the students to tell you how those arms and legs will look when the bear is turned around for them to see the back.

6. Using the overhead projector and in the form of a class discussion, work through *Rabbit Reversal* and *Designer Details*. Although students should attempt to find the correct pairs mentally, the teacher may want to make extra transparencies and cut out the shapes so that the answers from students can be tested.

CHALLENGE PAGES

Max's Hat Tricks
Make Max Reappear

7. Have students complete the Challenge Pages titled *Max's Hat Tricks* and *Make Max Reappear*.

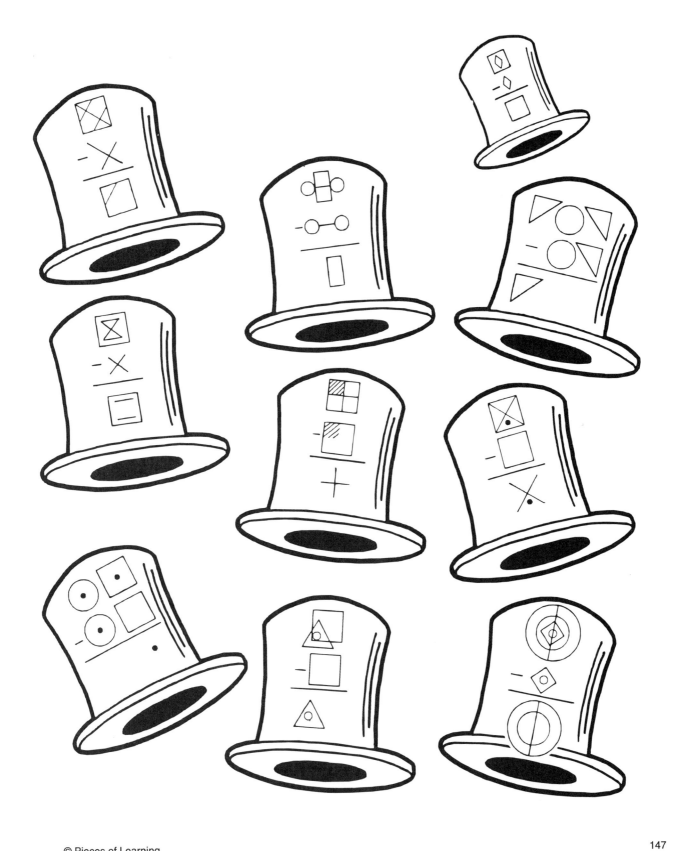

DIAGNOSTIC NOTES

During the whole class lesson, the teacher and observer are looking for students who have the ability to visualize the manipulations of the shapes. A checklist for the whole class lessons is provided. The following is a short summary of what to look for in student behaviors.

GRASPS CONCEPTS - Look for students who quickly see the perceptions presented. If they need to be shown the "trick," such as turning a pattern block, note those students who remember that "trick" and will try it in other situations.

SEES INTERRELATIONSHIP OF CLUES - Look for students who will use all available clues or ideas to try and figure out the pattern.

MANIPULATE SHAPES MENTALLY - Sometimes the teacher will be able to observe the students as they turn their heads or hands, trying to visualize or manipulate an object.

DEFERS JUDGMENT - These are the students who will wait to answer rather than jumping to a wrong conclusion.

INTUITIVELY SEES ANSWERS - Look for students who seem to intuitively understand the visual perceptions presented. They may have the correct answer without knowing how they got that answer.

Max's Hat Tricks and Make Max Reappear
Look for students who are able to correctly solve the puzzles and/or redraw Max.

NOTES

P E T S

Behavioral Checklist

Magician Thinking
(Visual/Spatial Perception)

List names of students as each behavior appears.

Add checkmarks after name if behavior is repeated.

Use a different color of ink or pencil for each whole group lesson.

Teacher _____
Grade: 1 ___ 2 ___ 3 ___

Dates of whole   1. _____
group instruction: 2. _____

GRASPS CONCEPTS VERY QUICKLY.	COMBINES VISUAL CLUES TO SOLVE PROBLEM -- *SEES INTERRELATIONSHIP OF CLUES.*
COMMENTS INDICATE AN ABILITY TO *MANIPULATE SHAPES MENTALLY*	GATHERS AND WEIGHS ALL INFORMATION BEFORE DECIDING ON AN ANSWER -- *DEFERS JUDGMENT.*
INTUITIVELY SEES ANSWERS WITHOUT INTERMEDIATE STEPS.	
PETS classwork indicates an outstanding ability to use this thinking skill.	The following student/s did not participate during the thinking skills lessons, but I see these behaviors during **regular class time**.

MAX THE MAGICIAN

Today was a very special day in Crystal Pond Woods. Dudley the Detective, Sybil the Scientist, Yolanda the Yarnspinner, Isabel the Inventor, and Jordan the Judge were on their way to the beach, along with all of the other animals from Crystal Pond Woods. Everyone was very excited because they knew that on this day they would see one of the best shows ever – Max the Magician was coming to the Woods.

Max is a rabbit, but a very unusual rabbit. Max was not born in Crystal Pond Woods like all the other animals. Max came out of a tall black hat, making Max a magical rabbit. His fur is white, his nose is pink, and he dresses in a beautifully patterned vest. He has a way of looking at things that seems magical.

Max studies the **shapes** and **patterns** that are all around him. Everyone quickly found seats as showtime approached. The lights dimmed, the audience hushed, and the curtain went up. The crowd cheered wildly as Max entered the stage. Max removed his tall, black hat and bowed deeply to the crowd. "Ladies and Gentlemen, welcome to the greatest show in the Woods."

Max set his tall, black hat on the table.

(At this time put the overhead transparency of "Max's Hatband" on the overhead projector.)

Max waved his right hand to the crowd and reached into his tall, black hat and pulled out a handful of brightly colored blocks.

(At this time put some overhead pattern blocks on the overhead projector and/or give students some pattern blocks.)

Pointing to the pattern on the hatband of his tall, black hat, Max challenged the crowd, "Can you use these special pattern blocks and make the pattern on my hatband?"

The crowd was excited. All the animals of Crystal Pond Woods love challenges and Max always provides special challenges.

(Allow students time to try to figure out the pattern. The pattern is a green triangle and the red trapezoid, but the red trapezoid is turned so the view of the trapezoid is actually a red rectangle.)

The tension in the crowd was great as the minutes passed. Finally, Rascal Raccoon yelled, "I figured it out!"

Rascal Raccoon joined Max the Magician on stage and shared his solution with the crowd.

"I did not immediately see the answer because I laid all of my blocks flat on the ground. I knew the green triangle was part of the pattern, but I did not see a red rectangle. Because the red trapezoid was the only red block, I picked up the red trapezoid and looked at it from all different sides. While doing this, I noticed that when I hold it like this, *(hold the red trapezoid so that the rectangle side is viewed)*, it shows a rectangle."

The crowd showed its appreciation of Rascal Raccoon's solution by cheering wildly.

"We want more! We want more!" yelled the crowd.

"Okay, okay," answered Max the Magician. "My assistant, the teacher, has many more tricks to show you."

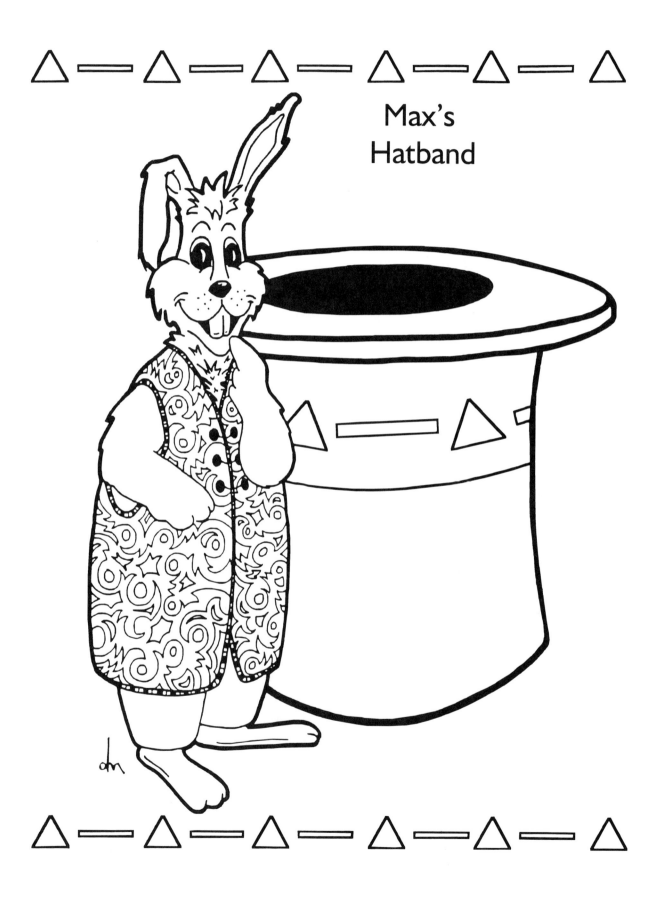

Max's
Hatband

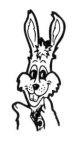

Max's Magic Hat

1. Cut out the 2 hat pieces along the solid lines.

2. Clip the edge of the hat top along all of the dotted lines. Fold the flaps out.

3. Roll the hat top and glue over the shaded area. Glue the top to the bottom around the shaded inner circle.

MAX
the
Magician

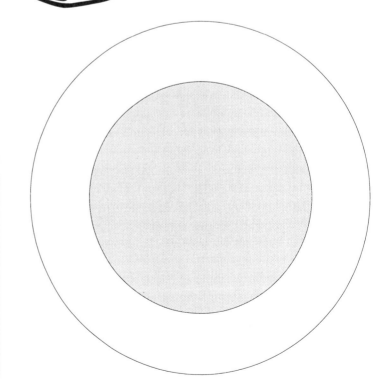

Rabbit Reversal

Which rabbit below is the real Max?

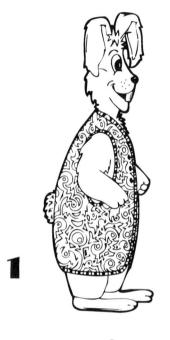

1

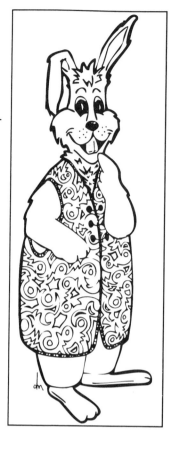

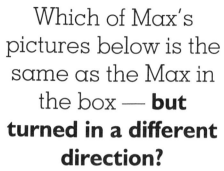

Which of Max's pictures below is the same as the Max in the box — but **turned in a different direction?**

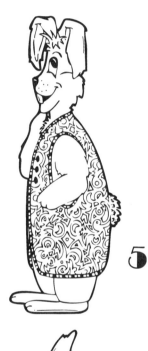

5

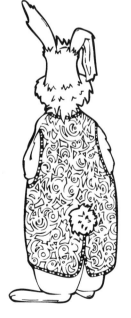

2

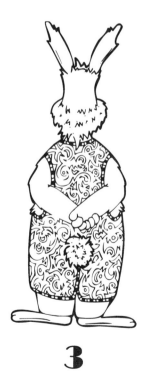

3

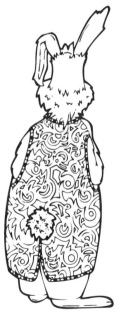

4

Designer Details

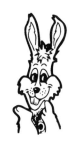

These designs are from Max's vest. Match each design with a letter to an identical shape with a number. Write the correct letter in each numbered shape.

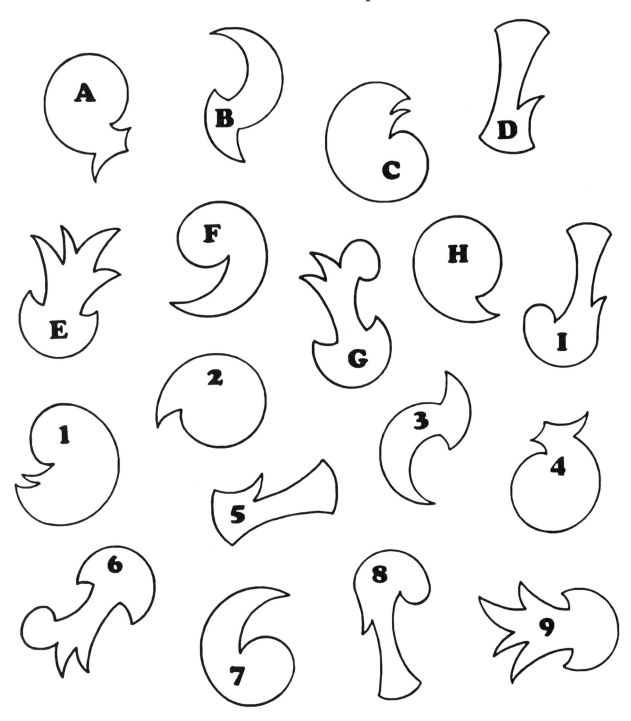

Name _____

Max's Hat Tricks

Subtract the figures in
each hat. Draw what's left.
Here's how:

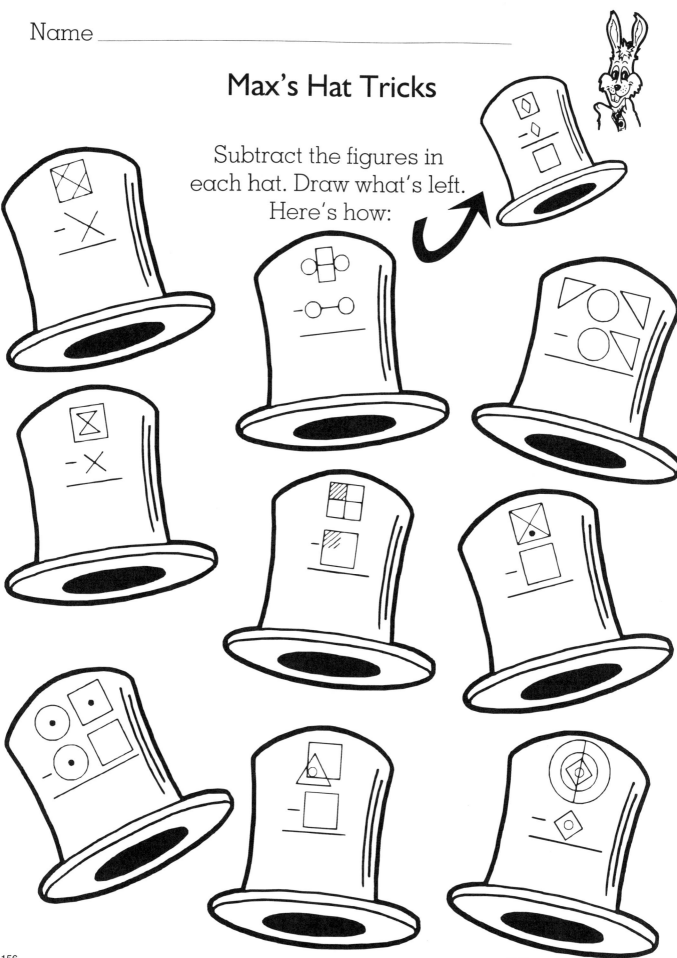

Name _____

Make Max Reappear

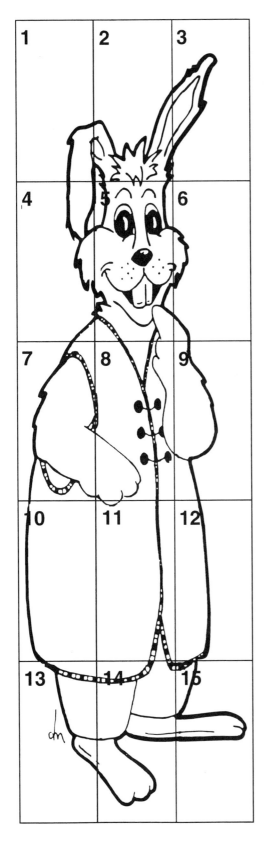

1	2	3
4	5	6
7	8	9
10	11	12
13	14	15

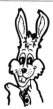

MAGICIAN THINKING
WHOLE CLASS
LESSON 2

PURPOSE

The purpose of this lesson is to review and reinforce the concepts presented in the previous lesson. Students will continue to practice their **visual/spatial perception** by analyzing patterns which repeat and extend, but are completely predictable. Students will also create original patterns using their visual high-level thinking.

TEACHER MATERIALS

— a set of manipulatives, such as Unifix cubes, for each student. If Unifix cubes are not available, a duplicated class set of *Pattern Panels* may be used
— a duplicated class set of *Hat Strings*
— Behavioral Checklist - *Magician Thinking*

STUDENT MATERIALS

— crayons or markers
— pencils
— scissors
— glue

LESSON PLAN

1. Review with students the concept of a *magician.* Magicians do not actually do magic. Instead they trick us by how we see or perceive things. During this unit, students are going to look at objects and study how they are perceived.

2. Each student will need a set of beads, Unifix Cubes, Cuisenaire rods, or other manipulatives suitable for creating patterns. *Pattern Panels* is provided to use instead of the manipulatives.

3. Using the manipulative, create a complicated, intricate pattern and ask the students to continue it. An example might be to create a stick of Unifix Cubes or a string of beads using the following pattern: yellow, blue, yellow, blue, blue, yellow, blue, blue, blue, yellow, blue, ...the students should use their own Unifix cubes to make the next ten steps in this pattern. The difficulty for the students is that they must begin their portion in the middle of the extending unit. Therefore, their stick or string should be blue, blue, blue, yellow, blue, blue, blue, blue, blue, yellow. Find someone with the correct response and add theirs to your own pattern and help the class to see why this response continues your pattern.

4. A second, more intricate pattern may be red, white, red, red, white, green, red, red, red, white, white, green, green, 4 reds, 3 whites, 3 greens. Ask students to continue the pattern by creating the next 10 steps. The correct response will be 5 reds, 4 whites, 1 green. Students may have difficulty stopping in the middle of a unit. Encourage them to only give you the next 10 steps.

5. Discuss how to find a pattern. How does one know where the pattern begins and ends? This second pattern seems to have some irrelevant information at the beginning. Elicit that there are patterns where the unit repeats and those where the unit extends. The essence of the pattern is that it is *predictable.* The students must disregard the blocks at the beginning and look for the beginning of the portion they can predict.

CHALLENGE PAGE

Hat Strings

6. Give students the Challenge Page titled *Hat Strings*. Tell the students that when they are finished they will cut the hats into five strips, horizontally across the page, and glue the strips end to end to create one long strip of hats.

7. Challenge the students to create a pattern to stump you by coloring the hats on the first four strips and leaving the last strip blank for the teacher to figure out.

DIAGNOSTIC NOTES

Look for students who can recognize and predict the pattern, even if it is in the middle of a unit. Also look for students who can design a complicated pattern which extends rather than repeats. Highest level thinkers will be able to create patterns which extend in a predictable manner, rather than patterns which simply repeat such as red, blue, red, blue no matter how long the unit.

NOTES

Name _____

Pattern Panels

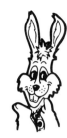

Hat Strings

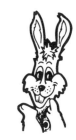

Create a pattern using these hats.

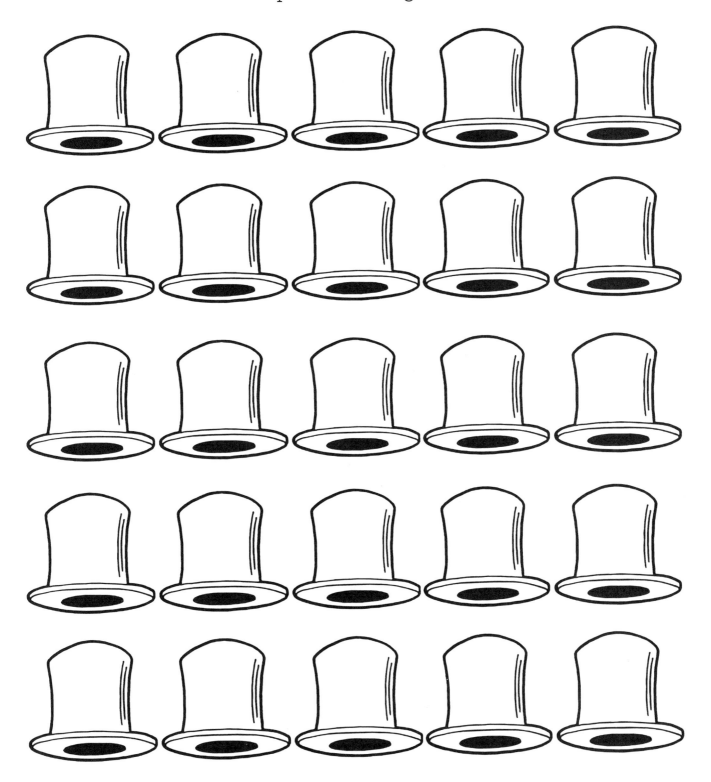

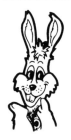

MAGICIAN THINKING
SMALL GROUP
LESSON 1

PURPOSE

The purpose of this lesson is to provide further visual/spatial problem solving through the **manipulation** of symmetrical shapes. Students will be challenged to arrange twenty-six pairs of symmetrical designs in a continuous pattern.

TEACHER MATERIALS

— a duplicated class set of *Max's Mirror Dominoes*. These should be cut out and laminated ahead of time and used repeatedly.

STUDENT MATERIALS

— scissors (only if students are cutting out their own dominoes)

LESSON PLAN

1. Students need to cut out *Max's Mirror Dominoes*. The students are to arrange the dominoes by choosing a domino to start with. Each end of the domino will have its mirror image on another domino. The students are to find the mirror image and begin making a domino train.

2. If students correctly match the dominoes, the last design placed will match the beginning of the train.

CHALLENGE PAGE

Look for students who find a strategy to solve the problem. For example, instead of looking for the "right design" one at a time, he or she matches pairs and then triplets as he or she finds them. With these multiple groups, longer trains can be made. The student quickly realizes that reversing the train is sometimes necessary to make a match. Look also for students who are able to quickly and accurately select the right design from the pile.

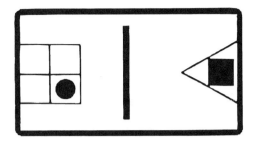

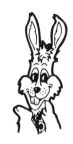

Max's Mirror Dominoes

Arrange the dominoes in a continuous pattern so that the design on the end of the last domino matches the beginning end of the first domino.

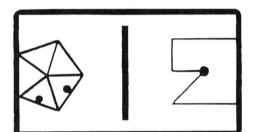

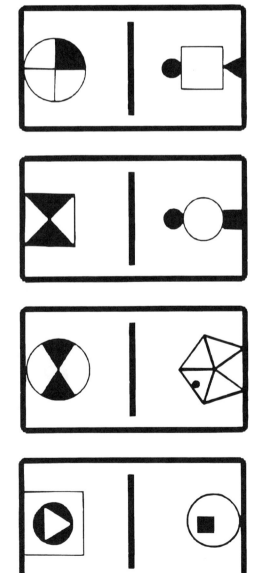

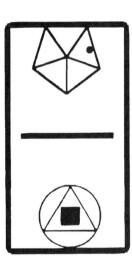

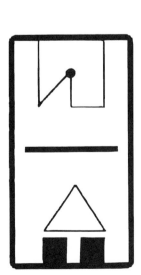

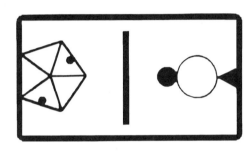

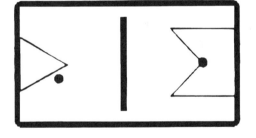

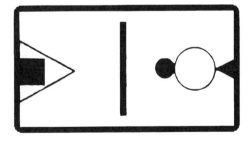

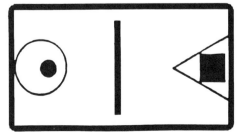

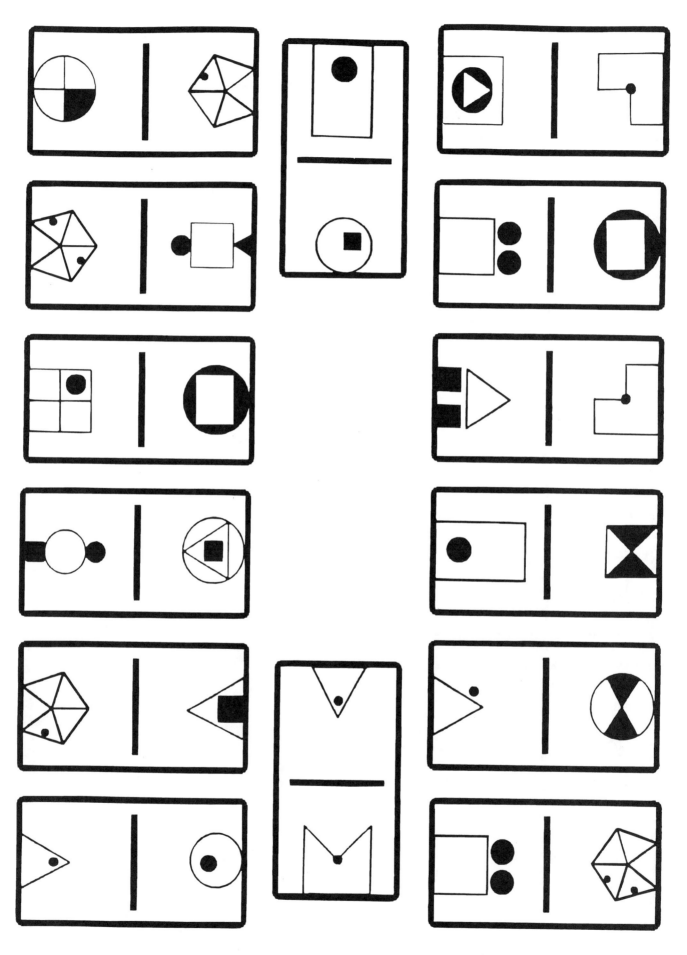

MAGICIAN THINKING
SMALL GROUP
LESSON 2

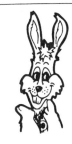

PURPOSE

The purpose of this lesson is to provide further visual/spatial problem solving through the **manipulation** of **tangrams**. As students rotate the tangrams to their correct positions, they solve the puzzles.

TEACHER MATERIALS

— a duplicated class set of *Max's Magic Tangrams*

STUDENT MATERIALS

— pencils
— scissors

LESSON PLAN

1. Give students the first page of *Max's Magic Tangrams.* The seven puzzle pieces are the tangram shapes and can be introduced to students if it is the first time they have used tangram. Students will need to cut out the pieces and put them together to make *Max the Magician*. Additional puzzles are included on the first page which require students to make two squares.

2. The tangram pieces can be used to solve the puzzles on the next two pages. If the pictures of Max the Magician interfere with the problem solving, have students turn the puzzle pieces over. If plastic tangrams are available, they can be used instead of the cut out pieces.

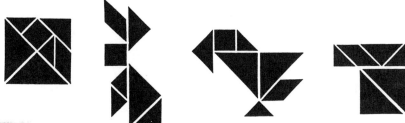

DIAGNOSTIC NOTES

Look for students who understand that some puzzle pieces can be used to cover the same area but in a different way. For example, the two small triangles can be used in place of the square. A capable student should be able to "see" these relationships and easily rotate or flip the shapes to solve the puzzles.

Max's Magic Tangrams

Max's vest has many pockets. In one very special pocket are his tangram pieces. Max makes puzzles with his tangrams. Use the puzzle pieces to solve Max's shapes and pictures.

Begin by putting Max back together again. This puzzle will make a rectangle.

Next, make a square with the two largest triangles. Now make a square the same size with all the other pieces.

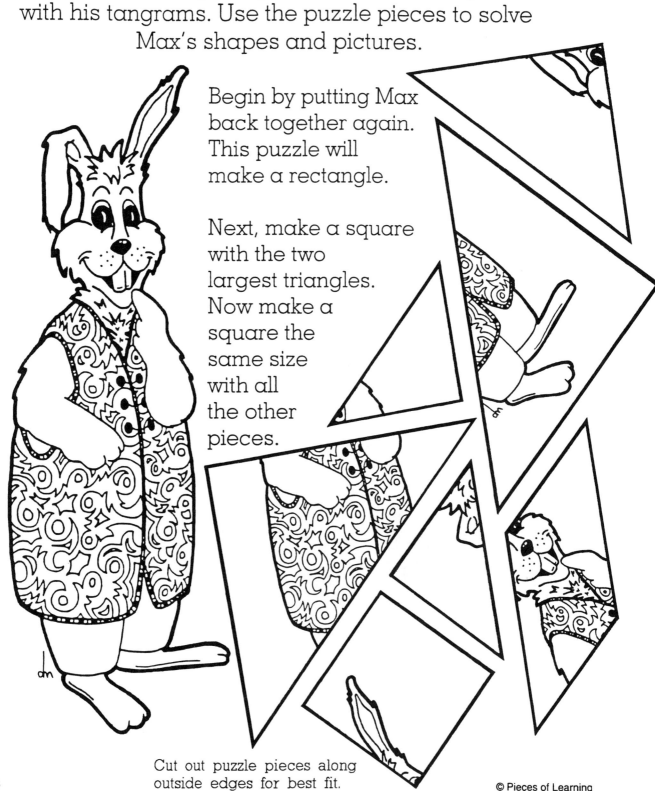

Cut out puzzle pieces along outside edges for best fit.

A Friend for Max

A Present for Max

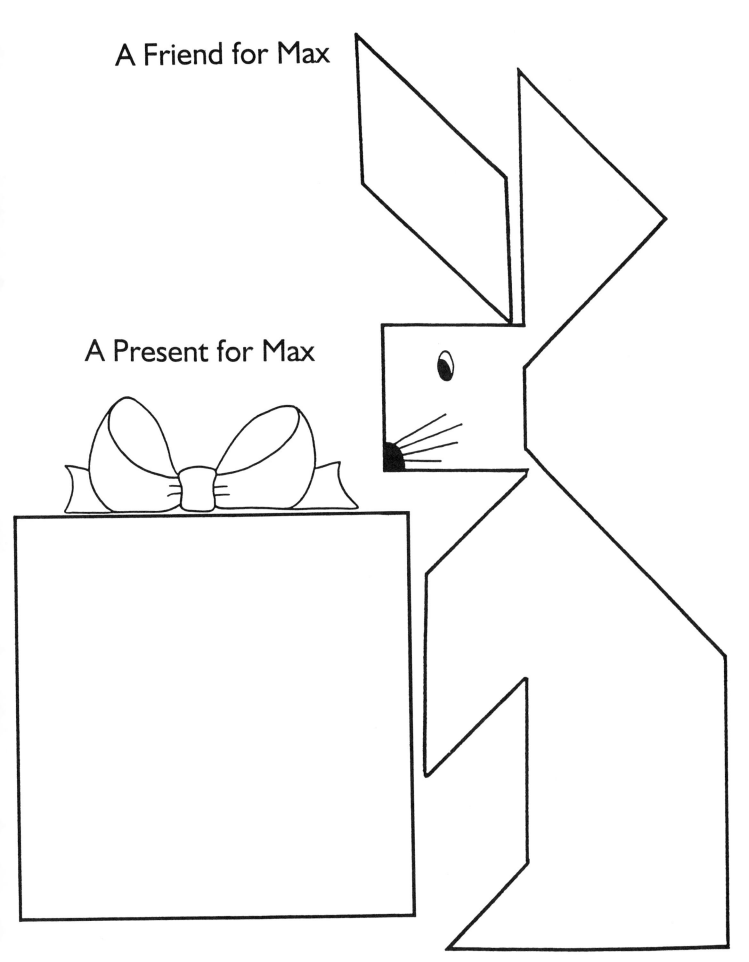

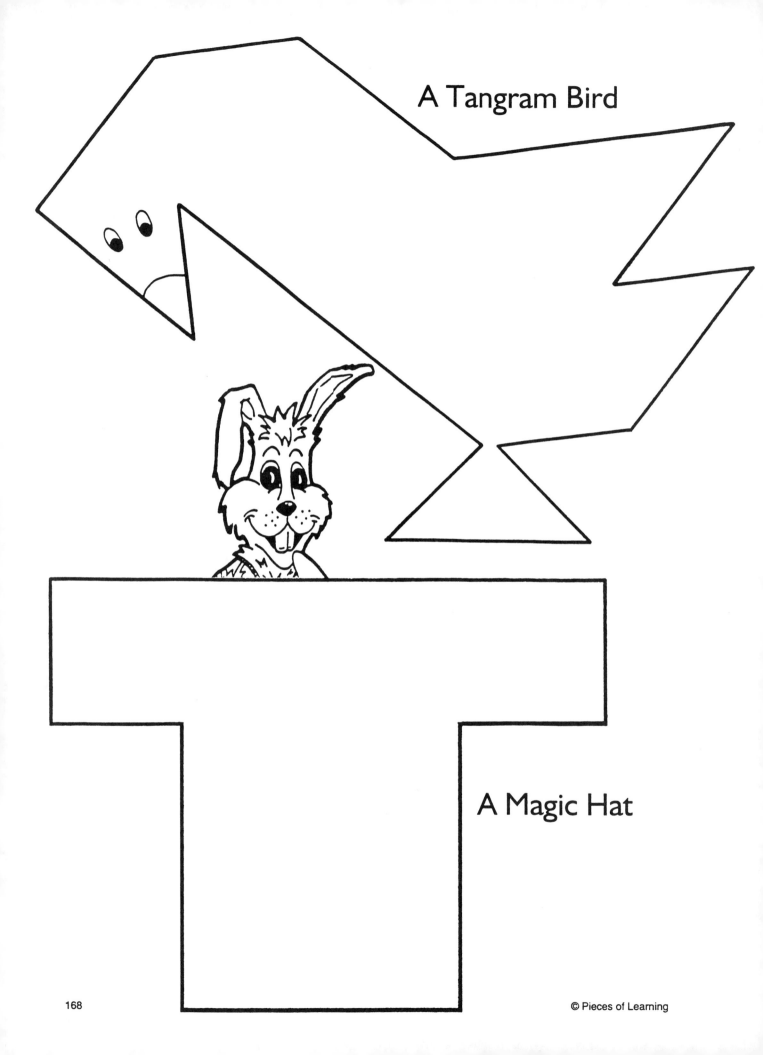

A Tangram Bird

A Magic Hat

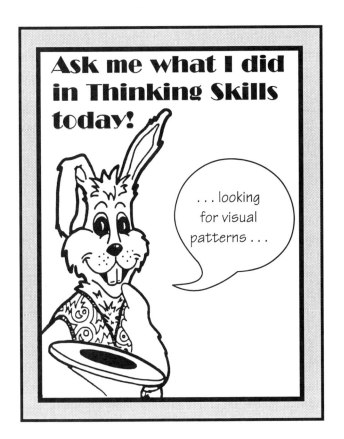

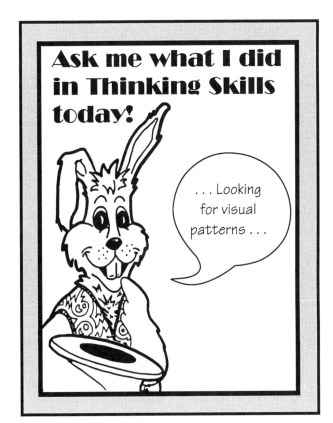

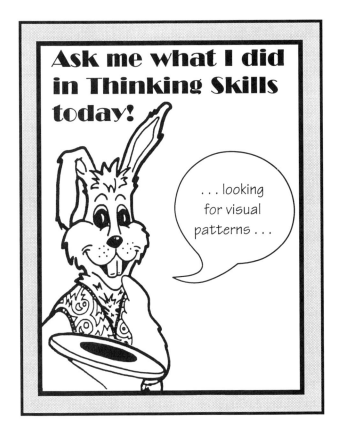

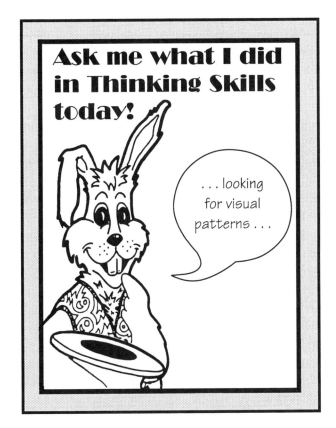

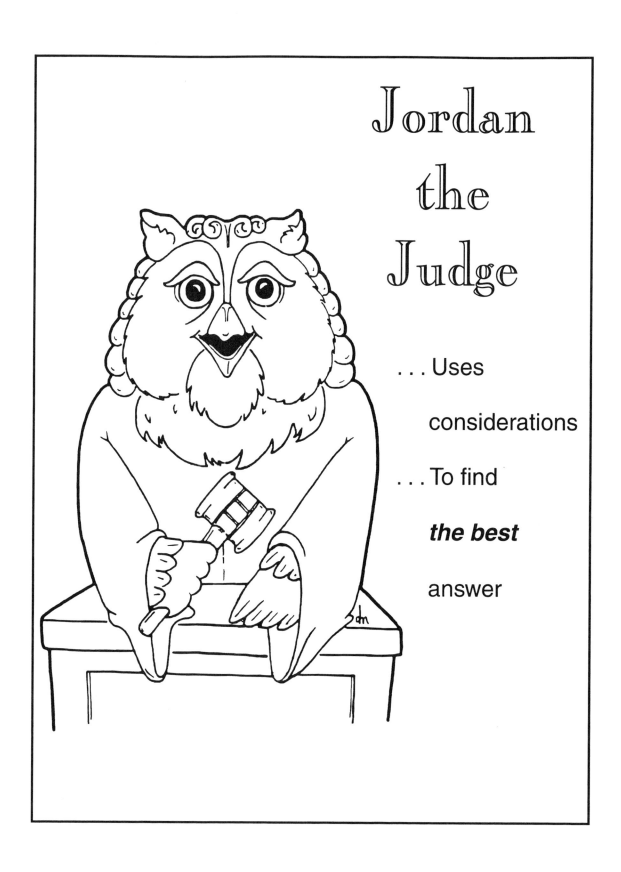

Jordan the Judge

. . . Uses

considerations

. . . To find

the best

answer

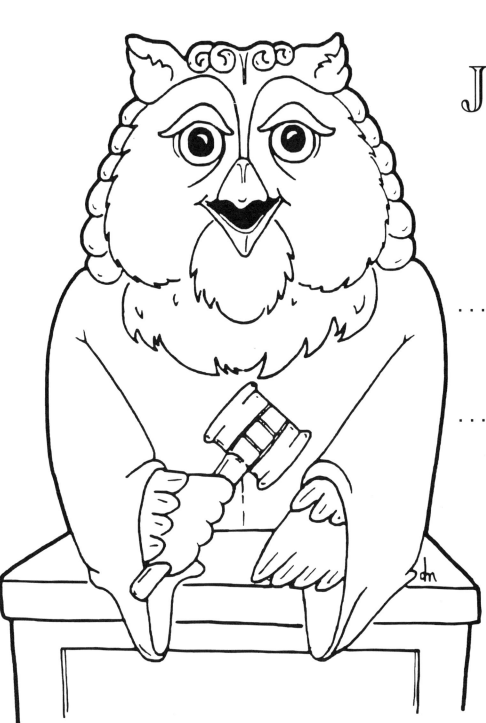

Jordan
the
Judge

. . . Uses

considerations

. . . To find

the best

answer

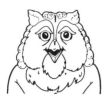

JUDGE THINKING
WHOLE CLASS
LESSON 1

PURPOSE

The purpose of this lesson is to introduce students to **evaluative thinking**. There are three types of evaluative thinking: criterion based evaluation, value judgements, and judicial evaluation. This lesson deals with criterion based evaluation. Through the story and character of Jordan the Judge, students will be encouraged to base decisions on factual criteria. The students will be instructed in the following concepts:

— Decisions are based on valid factual considerations, not on opinions.
— From amongst many choices, criteria can help guide students to the best answer, or to two or three "best" choices.

TEACHER MATERIALS

— one copy of the *Jordan the Judge* story
— an overhead transparency of the picture of *Jordan the Judge* and/or a class set of duplicated pictures for students to color
— a duplicated class set of *Jordan's Gavel* for students to cut out OR — pretzels and marshmallows for students to make gavels
— an overhead transparency of *Yolanda's List of Things to Buy*
— an overhead transparency of *What should we buy?*
— a duplicated class set of *A Pet For You*
— Behavioral Checklist - *Judge Thinking*

STUDENT MATERIALS

— crayons or markers
— pencil
— glue
— scissors

LESSON PLAN

1. Introduce students to the concept of a *judge*. Ask students if they know any judges. Give students the opportunity to describe what judges do. Discuss that judges are not only in a courtroom but there are also judges at contests.

2. Give students the picture of *Jordan the Judge* (page 171) or place a copy of *Jordan the Judge* (page 170) on the overhead projector.

3. Read the *Jordan the Judge* story.

4. Review with students that Jordan the Judge helps people make decisions by asking *"What are the considerations?"* When he has thought about all of the considerations, he bangs his gavel and announces his decision.

5. Have students cut out and color their gavels, the memory trigger for this unit. An alternative to the paper gavel is to have students make a gavel using big marshmallows and pretzels. They can quietly bang the gavels for the rest of the lesson.

6. As a class, work through *What should we buy?* on the overhead projector. Introduce the activity by pointing out that this time, in a pretend situation, the class has money to spend. As a class, the students will decide what to buy. With the class, brainstorm three items that might be bought for the class. Next list each item in the rectangular box with the corresponding number. As a class, brainstorm both "yes" considerations and "no" considerations. Discuss and reach consensus. Choose the best item to buy based on the considerations.

CHALLENGE PAGE

A Pet For You

7. Distribute the challenge page. The teacher may need to adjust the directions depending upon the reading and writing abilities of students. The ideal situation is to have students complete the challenge page independently while at school so the responses can be used in considering students for the small group sessions. If students do not have the skills to complete the worksheet independently, the teacher may need to read to students and work through the challenge page as a class.

DIAGNOSTIC NOTES

A checklist for the whole class lesson is provided. There is an overlap of characteristic behaviors and responses listed on the checklists of the six units. The following is a short summary of student behaviors and responses for the *Judge Thinking*.

GRASPS CONCEPTS VERY QUICKLY - Look for students who are able to quickly understand the concept of using considerations to eliminate choices and make a decision.

CAN LOGICALLY SUPPORT OPINIONS AND RESPONSES - Look for students who state opinions and can follow up their opinions with logical reasoning.

OFFERS UNIQUE SOLUTIONS AND/OR CONSIDERATIONS - Look for students who provide considerations that have not been previously stated. These considerations may even surprise the teacher.

DRAWS VALID CONCLUSIONS BASED UPON CONSIDERATIONS - Look for students who can accurately apply valid criteria in order to help narrow the field of many choices regardless of their own personal preferences.

SEE MORE THAN ONE VIEWPOINT - Look for students who are able to see the issue from another's viewpoint. This also shows strong potential. Especially notable are any students who are able to develop their own valid, factual criterion from the other viewpoint.

DISPLAYS A LONG ATTENTION SPAN - In addition to a long attention span, look for students who want to work on evaluative type activities. An enthusiasm toward this type of thinking usually indicates an ability to use it.

A Pet For You
Look for students who can create valid, factual criteria and apply them in the decision making process.

NOTES

P E T S

Behavioral Checklist

- - - - - - - - - - -

Judge Thinking
(Judge/Evaluative)

List names of students as each behavior appears.
    Add checkmarks after name if behavior is repeated.
    Use a different color of ink or pencil for each whole group lesson.

Teacher _____
Grade: 1 ___ 2 ___ 3 ___

Dates of whole   1. _____
group instruction: 2. _____

GRASPS CONCEPTS VERY QUICKLY.	*DRAWS VALID CONCLUSIONS BASED UPON CONSIDERATIONS* DEVELOPED IN THE LESSON
LOGICALLY SUPPORTS RESPONSES	*SEES MORE THAN ONE VIEWPOINT*
OFFERS UNIQUE SOLUTIONS AND/OR *CONSIDERATIONS*	*DISPLAYS LONG ATTENTION SPAN* -- WORKS EXERCISE DILIGENTLY TO THE END.
PETS classwork indicates an outstanding ability to use this thinking skill.	The following student/s did not participate during the thinking skills lessons, but I see these behaviors during **regular class time**.

JORDAN THE JUDGE

Yolanda the Yarnspinner and Rosalyn Robin were very excited one fine sunny day in Crystal Pond Woods. Yolanda had some extra money to spend. She had ten dollars to buy herself something special.

"Rosalyn Robin," sighed Yolanda. "I have so many things I want to buy. I can't decide how to spend my money. What do you think?"

"I think we need to go visit Jordan the Judge," suggested Rosalyn Robin. "He is always helping people with tough decisions so they make the **best choice.**"

Jordan is the Judge for Crystal Pond Woods. His courtroom is a very special place. He sits at the front of the courtroom, high above everyone else. He has a gavel that he uses to get the court's attention before announcing his decision.

Jordan always tells the animals how important it is to base their decisions on the facts. When one of the animals is having a hard time making a decision, Jordan asks the animal, "What are the **considerations?**" He listens to and thinks carefully about all the considerations. Then, after arriving at the best answer, Jordan the Judge bangs his gavel and announces his decision.

Yolanda and Rosalyn Robin arrived at Jordan's courtroom to discover that it was very busy. They had to wait awhile until it was their turn. Jordan the Judge then said, "Good afternoon, ladies, what can I help you with today?"

"Well, Jordan the Judge," began Yolanda. "I have ten dollars to spend, and I can't decide how to spend it. Here is a list of things I would like to buy."

Yolanda handed Jordan the Judge the list and he read it aloud.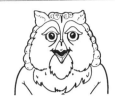

(Put a transparency of Yolanda's List on the overhead so students can follow along.)

"So, you would like a black purse, a computer, a fur coat, a gray hat, a vase, a book of poems, a pair of red mittens, an orange scarf, black earrings, a brown sweater, and a gray dress. Hmmm, so what are your considerations, Yolanda?"

"Well," said Yolanda, "I only have ten dollars."

"That helps," said Jordan the Judge. "We must eliminate all the items on your list that cost more than ten dollars."

(Discuss with students the items to be eliminated from the list because they cost more than ten dollars. Cross them off the list as students suggest. Be sure that students are only considering the cost at this time.)

"Okay, Yolanda," said Jordan the Judge in his superior voice. "Are there any other considerations?"

"Yes," replied Yolanda. "I want to buy something that will keep me warm in the winter."

"Well, well, that seems clear enough," said Jordan the Judge. "We must eliminate all the items on your list that are not items that can keep you warm."

(Now, discuss with students which items should be eliminated from the list based solely on this new consideration. Cross those items off the list.)

"Are there any further considerations?" Jordan the Judge asked Yolanda.

"Yes," answered Yolanda. "I love colorful words, and I want to buy something really colorful."

(Now discuss with students the items that should be eliminated based solely on the color criterion.)

"In that case, there are clearly two possibilities. You can buy the pair of red mittens or the orange scarf. Would there be another consideration to keep in mind?" inquired Jordan.

Rosalyn Robin looked at Yolanda with a smile on her face. "Of course there is!" she cried. "Yolanda is a spider and has eight arms!"

Jordan banged his gavel and proudly announced, "Then the decision seems very clear. Buy the orange scarf. Case dismissed!"

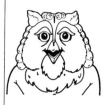

Yolanda's List
of
Things to Buy

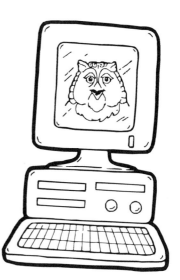

black purse

computer

fur coat

gray hat

vase

book of poems

pair of red mittens

orange scarf

black earrings

brown sweater

gray dress

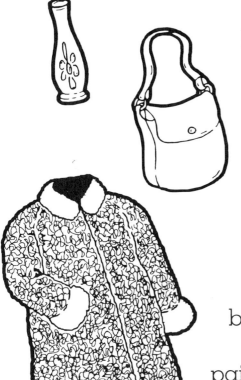

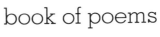

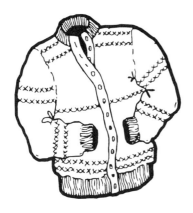

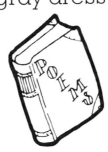

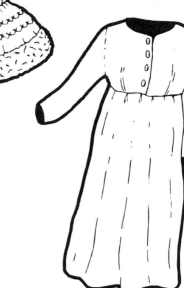

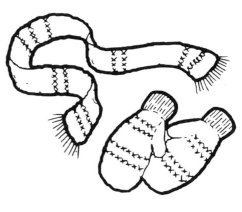

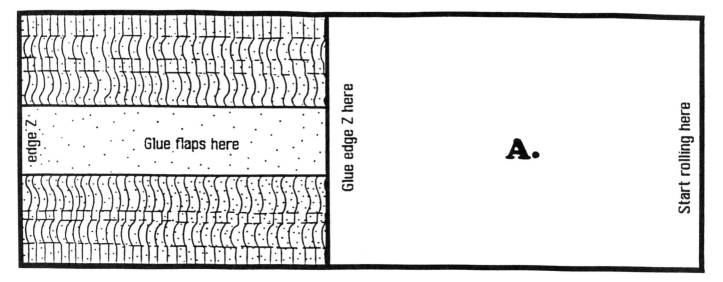

edge Z

Glue flaps here

Glue edge Z here

A.

Start rolling here

Jordan's Gavel

1. Cut out the 2 pieces (A, B) along the heavy, dark lines.

2. Roll up piece A and glue it closed (gluestick is best).

3. Fold piece B flat over and over along the dotted lines and glue it closed.

4. Fold out the flaps on piece B to form a Y.

5. Insert the roll into the Y formed by the flaps, lining up the flaps with the center channel. Overlap and glue the flaps around the roll.

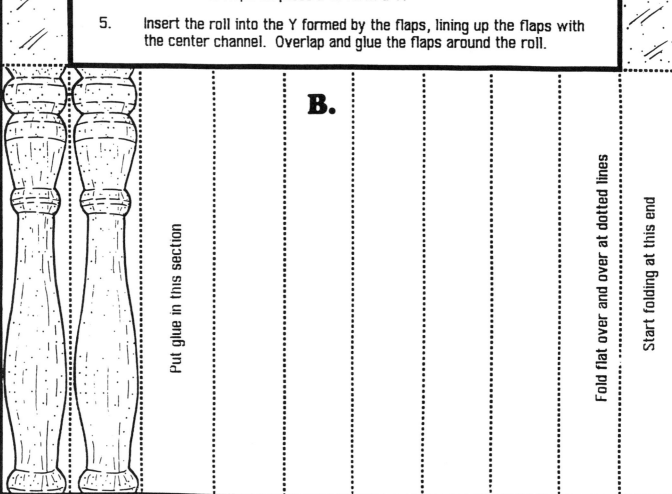

B.

Put glue in this section

Fold flat over and over at dotted lines

Start folding at this end

What should we buy?

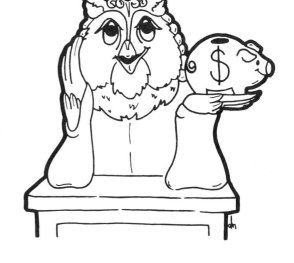

The classroom fund has grown for months. Now we are ready to buy something very special for the classroom — what will it be?

Brainstorm 3 things we might buy for the classroom:

1. _____ 2. _____

3. _____

But do we *really* want any of these wonderful things? Let's look at some "Yes" considerations and some "No" considerations.

1. [   ]

"Yes" considerations	"No" considerations
1.	1.
2.	2.
3.	3.

2.
┌───┐
│   │
└───┘

"Yes" considerations   "No" considerations

1.   1.

2.   2.

3.   3.

3.
┌───┐
│   │
└───┘

"Yes" considerations   "No" considerations

1.   1.

2.   2.

3.   3.

What's the best thing to spend our money on? Put a big star next to it!

Name _____

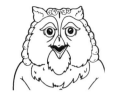

A Pet for You

Your parents have said you can choose a new pet!

Start with these 3 considerations. Read them carefully.
Check either YES or NO.

YES   **NO**

☐   Do I have a fence around my yard?   ☐

☐   Is anyone home during the day at my house?   ☐

☐   Is anyone at home allergic to pet hair?   ☐

What are some other things that you need to think about?
I want a pet that:

1. _____

2. _____

3. _____

Using these considerations, what's the BEST new pet
for you? Draw it.

My new pet
is a:

_____

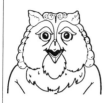

JUDGE THINKING
WHOLE CLASS
LESSON 2

PURPOSE

The purpose of this lesson is to introduce students to another way to **collect factual information** to use in the decision-making process. The students will collect facts from the story **Ira Sleeps Over** on a T-chart. Students will learn that:

— The T-chart is useful for collecting decision-making information.
— The number of facts and the importance of the facts on one side of the T-chart should help in the evaluative process.

TEACHER MATERIALS

— one copy of the story **Ira Sleeps Over** by Bernard Waber
— an overhead transparency of **Should Ira Take His Bear?**
— Behavioral Checklist - *Judge Thinking*

STUDENT MATERIALS

— crayons
— pencils
— scissors

LESSON PLAN

1. Review with students the key ideas related to *Jordan the Judge*. Remind students that a judge helps people make decisions by asking "What are the considerations?" When a judge has thought about all of the *considerations,* he/she bangs the gavel and announces the best solution.

2. Introduce the story **Ira Sleeps Over** by explaining to students that they are going to hear a story about Ira. Ira has an important decision to make. As the story is read, the class will make a list of the considerations Ira needs to think about to help him make his decision. Explain to students that in order to organize the considerations, they are going to use a T-chart. It is called a T-chart because of its shape. Show students the overhead transparency of *Should Ira Take His Bear?*

3. Read the story to the students, pointing out Ira's dilemma of whether or not to take his teddy bear when his friend invites him to sleep over. As the different criteria are introduced in the story, list them on the overhead transparency, *Should Ira Take His Bear?* As the story gives pertinent information, stop and ask students whether this new fact is a reason why Ira should or should not take his teddy bear to Reggie's house.

On the "Yes" side:
1. Ira has never slept without his teddy before.
2. Reggie is planning to tell scary ghost stories.
3. Reggie has his own bear, and it has a baby name, too.

On the "No" side:
1. Reggie will laugh and say Ira is a baby.
2. Reggie will laugh and say "Tah-Tah" is a baby name.

4. Discuss with students the T-chart. Ask students which side has more reasons. Discuss with students whether or not any of the considerations is more important than the others. When making a decision, some considerations are more important than others and therefore carry more weight. In the case of Ira, not only were there more "Yes" considerations, but the most important consideration, #3, is also on the "Yes" side. Ira should definitely have chosen to take his teddy bear, and Jordan the Judge is satisfied that Ira has decided wisely.

CHALLENGE PAGE

Brainstorming Considerations

5. Distribute the Challenge Page *Brainstorming Considerations.*

DIAGNOSTIC NOTES

A checklist for the whole class lesson is provided. There is an overlap of characteristic behaviors and responses listed on the checklists of the six units. The following is a short summary of students' behaviors and responses for the Judge Thinking Unit.

GRASPS CONCEPTS VERY QUICKLY - Look for students who can determine which facts from the story are pertinent in Ira's decision making and on which side of the T-chart they belong.

CAN LOGICALLY SUPPORT OPINIONS AND RESPONSES - Look for students who state opinions and can follow up their opinions with logical reasoning.

OFFERS UNIQUE SOLUTIONS AND/OR CONSIDERATIONS - Look for students who offer considerations related to, but not directly from, the story.

DRAWS VALID CONCLUSIONS BASED UPON CONSIDERATIONS - Look for students who show strong potential in evaluative thinking. They will be able to see that the T-chart information comprises the criteria for the decision-making process, regardless of their own personal feeling towards teddy bears.

SEES MORE THAN ONE VIEWPOINT - Look for students who are able to see the issue from another's perspective. These students may also understand how the decision may be different depending on the character making the decision.

DISPLAYS A LONG ATTENTION SPAN - In addition to a long attention span, look for students who want to work on evaluative type activities. An enthusiasm towards this type of thinking usually indicates an ability to use it.

NOTES

Should Ira Take His Bear?

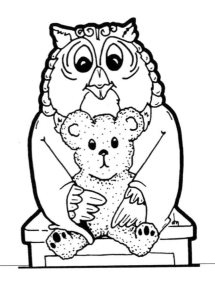

What are the considerations?

take the bear	leave the bear

Name _____

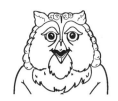

Brainstorming Considerations

What do you think about, or consider, when you have to make a decision? What questions do you ask yourself? What considerations help you make the <u>best</u> choice?

List the considerations you think would be important to you if you had to make these 3 decisions:

1. Shall I buy this pair of gym shoes?

1. _____

   _____

2. _____

   _____

3. _____

   _____

4. _____

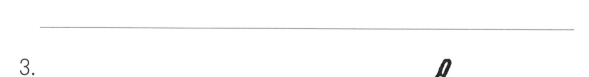

Name _____

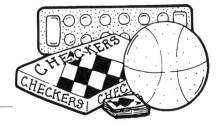

2. What game do I want to play?

   1. _____

   2. _____

   3. _____

   4. _____

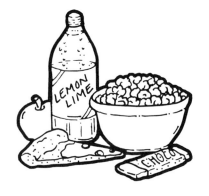

3. What shall I eat for a snack?

   1. _____

_____

   2. _____

_____

   3. _____

_____

   4. _____

_____

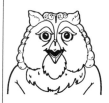

JUDGE THINKING
SMALL GROUP
LESSON 1

PURPOSE

The purpose of this lesson is to reinforce and extend the evaluative concepts presented in class. Students will be **applying factual criteria** in making decisions and supporting their points of view.

TEACHER MATERIALS

— a duplicated class set of *Jordan's Notable Necessities*
— a class set of *Jordan's Notable Necessities Cards* which have been cut out, laminated, and are ready to use

STUDENT MATERIALS

— pencils

LESSON PLAN

1. Review with students the characteristics of evaluative thinking. In order to make the best decision, a judge will ask, "What are the considerations?" These considerations should be based on *factual information.*

2. It is helpful to have the decks of cards colored, mounted on index cards and possibly laminated.

3. Choose one of the decks to demonstrate the lesson with the entire group. Spread the eight cards on the table and the instruction card from *Jordan's Notable Necessities.*

4. In the form of a class discussion, ask students to select the six items they need most to accomplish the task. Allow students time to discuss each item and its relevance to the task. When the group has selected six items, have them prioritize the cards, ranking the items from most important to least important. Encourage factual criteria as support for their choices, and allow good-natured debate and disagreement. Encourage students to support their ideas and persuade the group toward their points of view. Throughout this activity, it is the criteria which are important, not the actual selections. The teacher should never allow his or her own opinion to enter into the discussion; rather, students' points of view should be validated as long as their support and criteria are reasonable.

5. After the entire group has participated in the guided evaluative activity, divide the group into two smaller groups and give each group another set of the cards. Groups will

have different task cards at this point. Ask each group to independently work through the same evaluative task as before, but without any teacher guidance. The teacher's role is simply to monitor discussions and listen for students who are capable of making evaluations based on sound factual criteria.

DIAGNOSTIC NOTES

Look for students who can apply their own factual criteria, make valid evaluations and support their points of view. Look for students who are able to see other viewpoints.

NOTES

Jordan's Notable Necessities

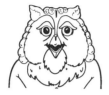

Using the appropriate deck of cards, select and rate the 6 most needed items to accomplish these 3 tasks.

Build a Doghouse

1. Select the 6 items from the set of 8 that you feel are most needed to build a doghouse.

2. Rank these 6 items from most important to least important.

3. Explain your choices and rating.

Bake a Cake

1. Select the 6 items from the set of 8 that you feel are most needed to bake a cake.

2. Rank these 6 items from most important to least important.

3. Explain your choices and rating.

Paint a Picture

1. Select the 6 items from the set of 8 that you feel are most needed to paint a picture.

2. Rank these 6 items from most important to least important.

3. Explain your choices and rating.

Paint a Picture Card Set

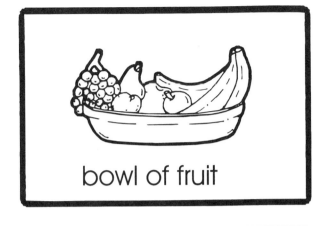
bowl of fruit

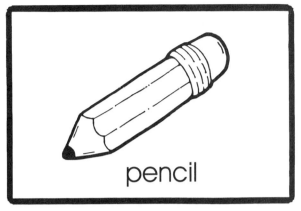
pencil

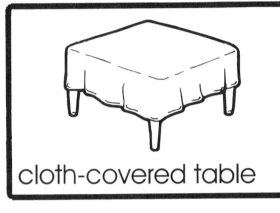
cloth-covered table

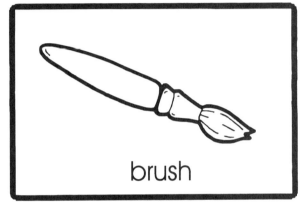
brush

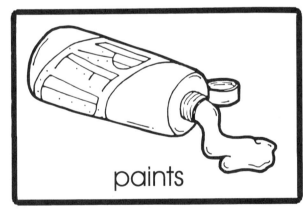
paints

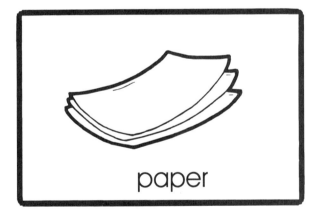
paper

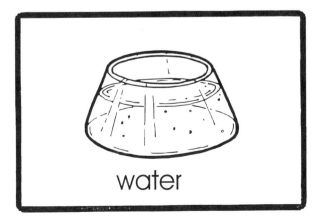
water

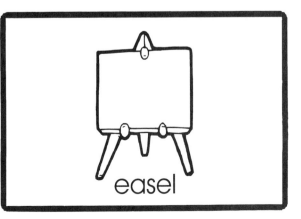
easel

Build a Doghouse Card Set

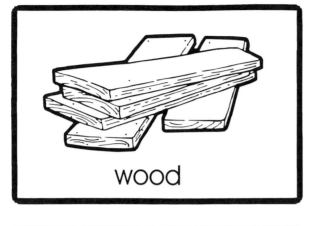

wood

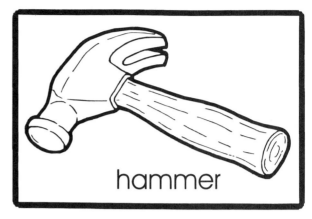

hammer

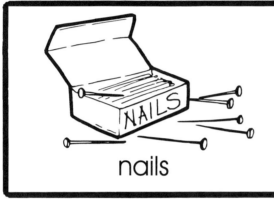

nails

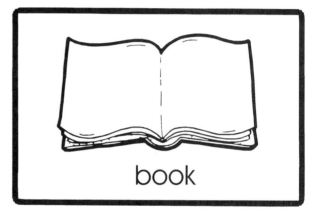

book

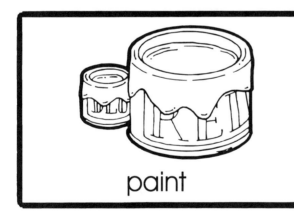

paint

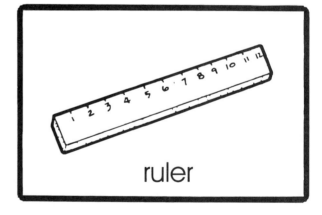

ruler

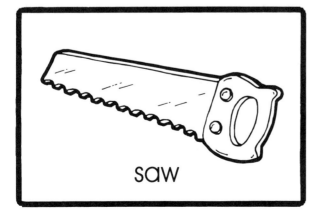

saw

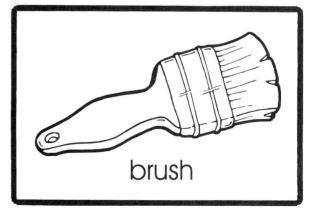

brush

Bake a Cake Card Set

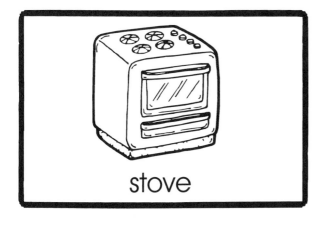

stove

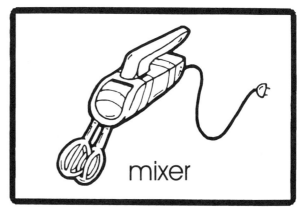

mixer

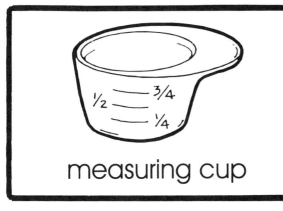

measuring cup

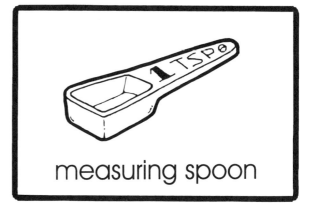

measuring spoon

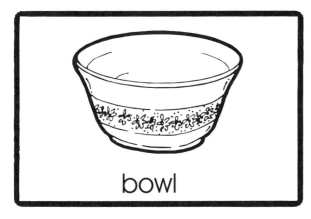

bowl

mixing spoon

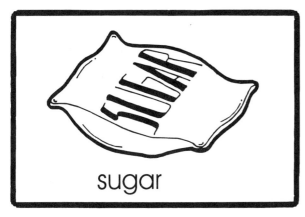

sugar

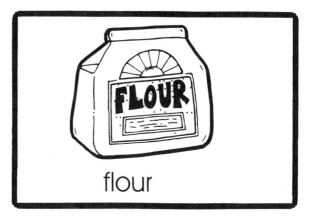

flour

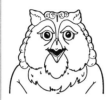

JUDGE THINKING
SMALL GROUP
LESSON 2

PURPOSE

The purpose of this lesson is to reinforce the use of criteria when making decisions. Students will be supporting their choices with specific criteria.

TEACHER MATERIALS

— one copy of *A Very Buggy BZZZZZness* chart for each student
— one copy of *A Very Buggy BZZZZZness* bugs for each student
— an 8.5" x 11" sheet of white paper for each student
— an 11" x17" sheet of colored construction paper for each student

STUDENT MATERIALS

— crayons or markers
— pencils
— scissors
— glue

LESSON PLAN

1. Review the characteristics of **thinking like a judge**. Explain to students that in this lesson they are going to use considerations about bugs to decide what kinds of bugs are going to live in the world.

2. Brainstorm all the types of bugs students can think of. Record the list of bugs.

The term "bugs" is used here deliberately to allow students to include insects (3 body parts, 6 legs), arachnids (such as spiders, daddy longlegs, mites, and ticks that have 2 body parts and 8 legs), and some arthropods (such as centipedes and millipedes that have long multi-segmented bodies and many legs.) Insects are classified according to the physical characteristics of the adult form which explains why many-legged caterpillars are still considered to be insects. Slugs (terrestrial mollusks) and worms (annelids) would not be included.

3. Brainstorm the good things and bad things about bugs. Record this list, too.

Some specific points about bugs included in this lesson:

Little black ants	most abundant of all land animals great food source for birds and other animals destroy other pests and insects scavenge human food some specialized ants: harvest seeds, raise fungus for good, eat leaves cut from plants, tunnel in wood, kill and eat nesting birds
Swallowtail butterflies	largest and most gorgeous butterfly feed on leaves
Ground beetles	colorful known as caterpillar hunters eat lots of pests
House flies	feed by lapping up liquids spread disease
Orb weaver spiders	eat insects make a spiraling orb-shaped web; each night, the old web is replaced with a new one; spun in complete darkness by touch alone; takes about one hour; it will hold 4000 times the spider's own weight; uses about 63 feet of silk each kind of orb weaver spider spins its own kind of web; from the moment it leaves its egg it knows how to spin a certain pattern
Honey bees	most important pollinator make honey use bee "language" — a complex direction-giving dance
Dragonflies	eat flying insects including mosquitoes
Crickets	eat plants, pests, blankets, sweaters, baskets make chirping sounds by rubbing wings together
Ladybug beetles	eat aphids and other pests
Firefly beetles	create light through a chemical reaction in abdomen blink light to attract a mate

4. Give students the worksheet *A Very Buggy BUZZZZZness* chart. Each student is to go through the list of bugs and in the narrow check boxes check "yes" for each bug to be included or "no" for each bug not to be included in the student's world. The

consideration on which this decision is based for each bug is then written in the large box beside each check. Students may add additional considerations.

5. Have students draw a picture of the world or some special place in the world on the white piece of paper. Give each student a copy of *A Very Buggy BUZZZZZness* bugs. Only the bugs that were checked "yes" are to be cut out and added to the student's drawing.

6. Have students fold their sheets of construction paper in half. On the inside halves, they should glue their *A Very Buggy BUZZZZZness* chart and drawing. On the outside of this construction paper folder, have students title their work and write their names.

DIAGNOSTIC NOTES

Look for students who can generate and understand factual considerations, can apply them to make valid choices, and can support their points of view. Watch for a complexity of thought that demonstrates the capacity to see other points of view, which recognizes that weighing a variety of factors may be a never-ending process, and that addresses the importance of ecological interrelationships.

NOTES

Name _____

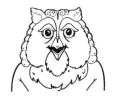

A Very Buggy Buzzzzzness

Wow! You can choose what bugs will live in your world!

What bugs will there be? Why? What are your considerations?

BUGS	Yes	✔	No	✔
Black Ants				
Swallowtail Butterflies				
Ground Beetles				
House Flies				
Orb Weaver Spiders				
Honey Bees				
Dragonflies				
Crickets				
Ladybug Beetles				
Fireflies				

Name _____

A Very Buggy Buzzzzzness!

Cut out the
bugs you want
in your world.

Glue them
into your picture.

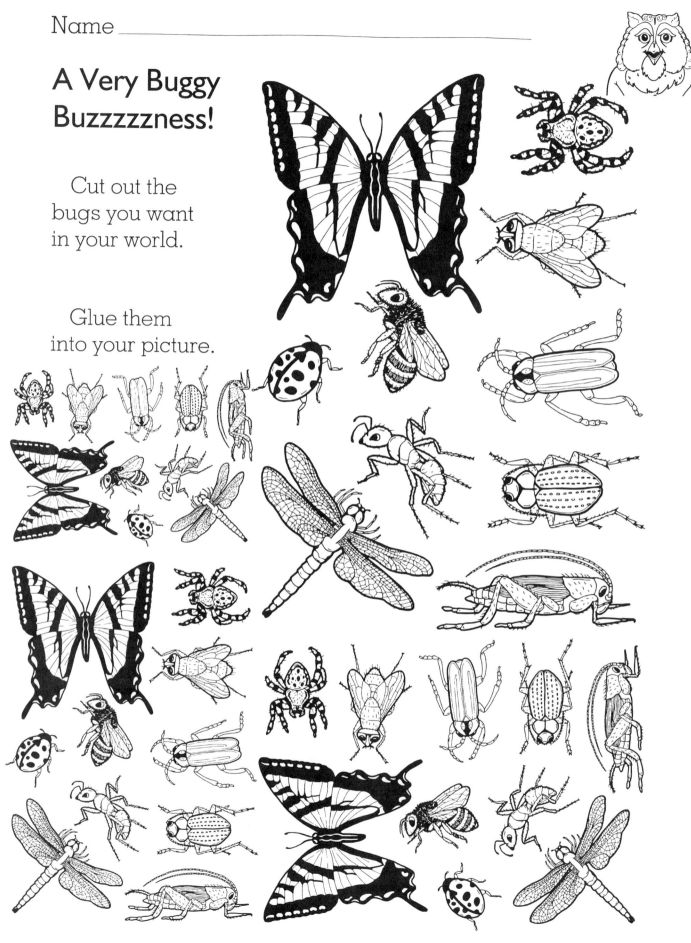

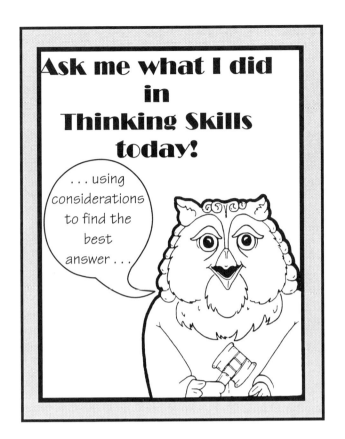

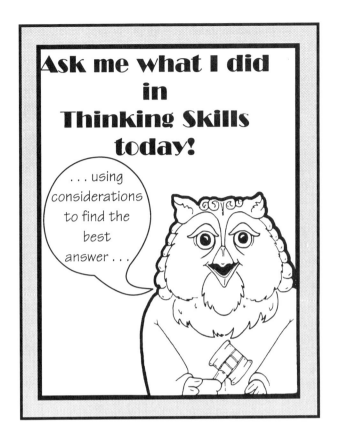

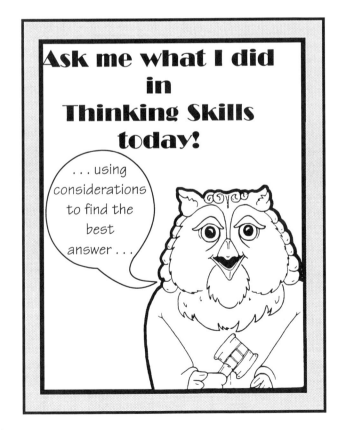

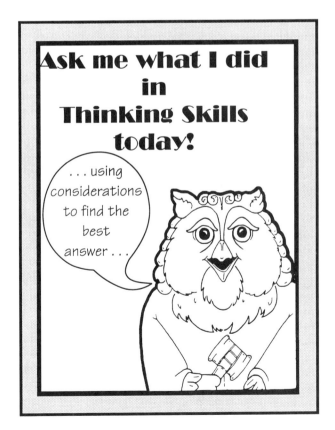

Convergent / Deductive Thinking

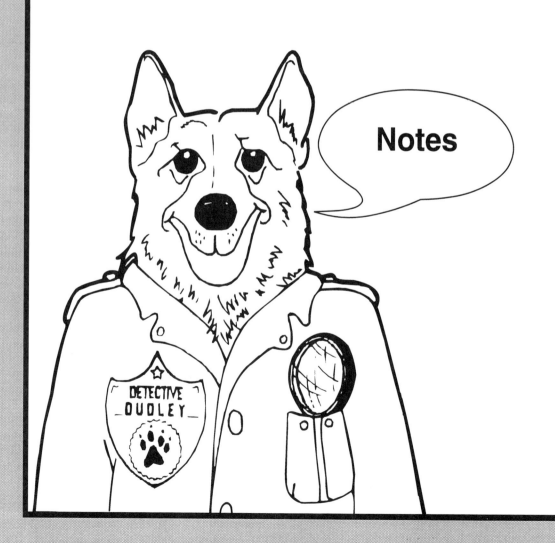

Divergent / Inventive Thinking

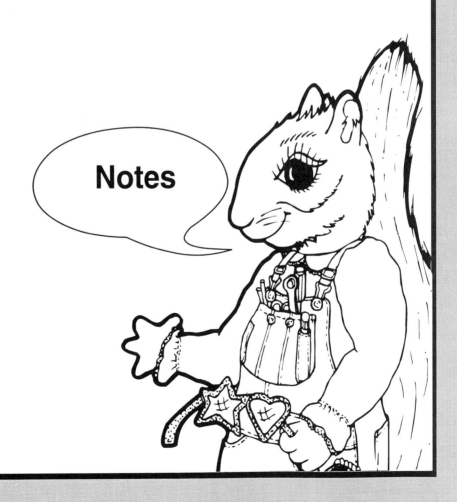

Convergent / Analytical Thinking

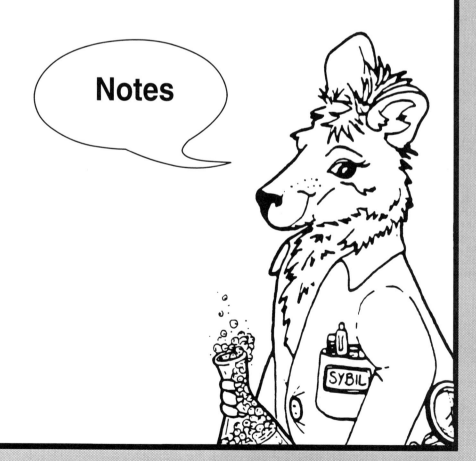

Divergent / Creative Thinking

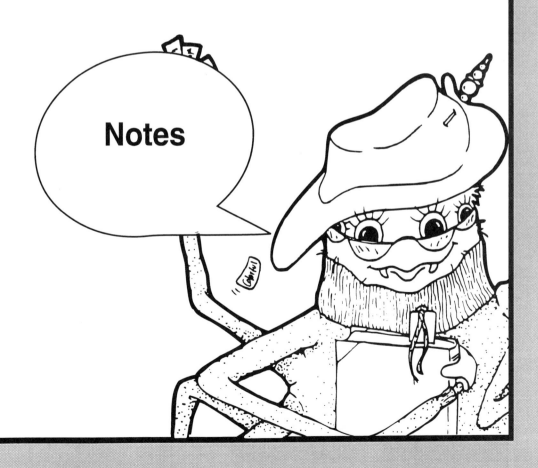

Visual / Spatial
Perception

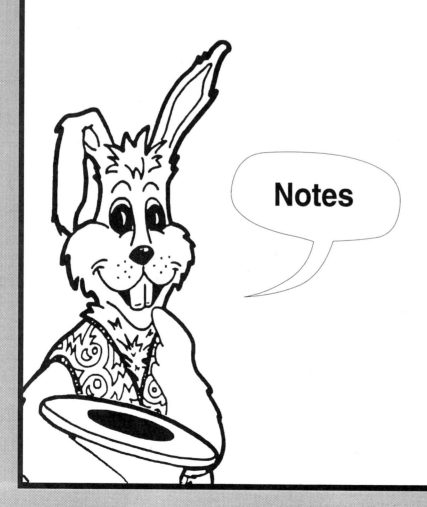

Evaluative
Thinking

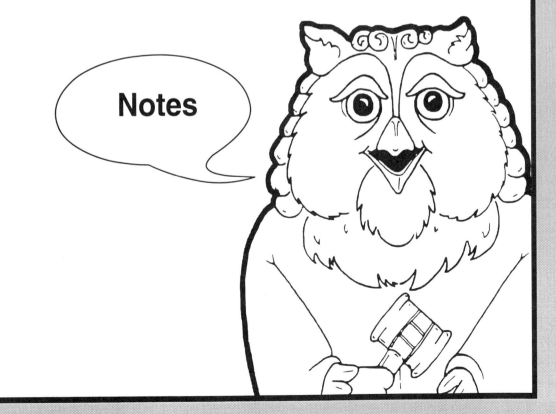